PROJECT 2000:
THE TEACHERS SPEAK

PROJECT 2000:
THE TEACHERS SPEAK

Innovations in the Nursing Curriculum

Edited by
Oliver Slevin and Mike Buckenham

Campion Press

British Library Cataloguing-in-Publication Data

Project 2000: the teachers speak.
I. Slevin, O. D'A II. Buckenham, M. A.
610.730941

ISBN 1-873732-00-7

First published 1992 by
Campion Press Ltd,
384 Lanark Road,
Edinburgh EH13 0LX

Acknowledgements
We are grateful to the National Board for Nursing, Midwifery and
Health Visiting for Northern Ireland, and Sage Publishing, USA,
for permission to reproduce the tables on pages 33 and 37.

Cover design:
Artisan Graphics, Edinburgh

Typesetting:
Word Power, Auchencrow

Printed and bound by
The Alden Press, Oxford.

Contents

The Contributors

Mike Buckenham is Principal of Cheshire College of Health Care Studies.

Philip Cheung is Principal of the Health Services Initiatives and Development Unit, Queen's College, Glasgow.

Gaye Heathcote is Reader in Health Studies and Director of the Health Research and Development Unit at Crewe & Alsager College of Higher Education.

Geoff Hunt is the Director of the National Centre for Nursing and Midwifery Ethics.

Janet James is a Senior Teacher in North Trent College of Nursing and Midwifery.

David Jones is Principal of North Trent College of Nursing and Midwifery.

Carol Kirby is a Nurse Teacher in the Western Area College of Nursing, Northern Ireland.

Patricia Scott is a Professor of Nursing at the University of Ulster.

Oliver Slevin is Principal Professional Officer at the National Board for Nursing, Midwifery and Health Visiting for Northern Ireland.

Elizabeth Sweet is the Head of the Common Foundation Programme at Cheshire College of Health Care Studies.

Geoffrey Watts is Vice Principal of Cheshire College of Health Care Studies.

Preface

Project 2000: The Teachers Speak is the outcome of a series of seminars held in the United Kingdom in the summer of 1991. These seminars, sponsored by the Campion Press and entitled 'Project 2000: Resourcing the Curriculum', were received positively. It became clear at these seminars that teachers of nursing are now facing the most significant changes this century. Much has been written about overall strategy. A number of major research studies on the changes are already under way. However, as teachers and others prepare for and implement Project 2000 there is a need to reflect on this major innovation and share experiences. As a consequence it was felt that the four papers delivered at the seminars should be made more widely available. This book includes the four original papers and seven others from invited authors. Each contributor is an educationalist involved in some way with the new Project 2000 courses.

Project 2000: A New Preparation for Practice (UKCC, 1986) represented a major change in nurse education and professional nursing structures in the United Kingdom. The preparation for a new single-level practitioner who would be knowledgeable in his/her practice across a wide range of professional activities represented a major shift in emphasis. The new 'knowledgeable doer' would be capable of competent practice in hospital *and* community settings. He/she would be orientated toward and competent in health promotion and the prevention of ill-health as well as in care of the sick and disabled. Educational aspirations previously only contained in the most progressive programmes were to become the norm. Change-orientation; the capacity to learn and problem-solve in rapidly changing health care situations; the capacity for critical thinking and reflective practice; a move away from a narrow apprenticeship and training model to a more holistic educational approach in which students are supernumerary and the programme is education-led in all its aspects; a commitment to establishing practice on a sound knowledge base, with an emphasis on research-based practice and a commitment to integrating theory and practice in a care-orientated praxis: all these aspirations entailed changes which could quite reasonably be termed revolutionary in their impact on nurse education. When the proposals in the UKCC's New Preparation for Practice document were given government approval at the end of the 1980s, those involved in nurse education were faced with the most radical changes in the nursing curriculum since the Nightingale era.

The aforementioned developments in themselves represented far-reaching changes in our educational system. But when the UKCC decided, quite rightly, that the new curriculum represented a significant increase in the pace and level of study and ruled that all Project 2000 programmes should lead to the award of at least a higher education diploma, the changes were at once even more profound. The requirement for a higher education award necessitated links with the higher education sector which could range from course validation links right through to integration of nursing colleges into higher education institutions. Nurse teachers and their students found themselves faced not only with a new and radically different curriculum, but with functioning at a higher education level and within a higher education culture.

The first Project 2000 courses began in England in 1989. Since then the implementation process has proceeded across the United Kingdom. Further courses have commenced in England and Wales during 1990-1992. In Northern Ireland full implementation of the Project took place in all nursing colleges between October 1990 and May 1991 and developments are now in hand to integrate all nursing colleges into the universities in Northern Ireland, possibly by the mid-1990s. New Project courses are now set to commence in Scotland. In the course of designing and implementing the new curricula educators are involved in much creative thinking – fundamental educational philosophies are being reviewed, new curriculum models are being developed, methods of curriculum delivery not previously utilised are being implemented. And, perhaps more importantly, those who have already implemented the new programmes have gained the most useful experience, have already experienced successes and failures and resolved problems others have yet to face. There is a real need for dialogue and a sharing of experiences. This is already being facilitated by the contributions in professional journals, informal networks and information coming to hand from the first evaluative research projects. This book represents a further attempt to contribute to the sharing of information and dialogue on the new system of education.

Each of the contributors has been involved with the Project 2000 initiative in some way. They come from a variety of nursing and non-nursing backgrounds and in each case their contribution reflects their experience and background. The editors have taken as their remit the task of facilitating each author in presenting his/her contribution in accordance with his/her particular perspective or disciplinary orientation. No attempt was made to impose a common form or style and no attempt was made to hold contributors to a rigid structure. In this sense the book is seen as a vehicle to allow authors to share their experiences and views in a style which they feel is most appropriate. The readers will therefore not find in this text a structured and comprehensive treatment of the Project 2000 initiative; nor will they find a 'work manual' for Project 2000 implementation. Instead, what they find here is a collection of what are in essence essays by educators who have something to say about the new programmes in terms of their ideas, philosophies and experiences.

The collection commences in Chapter 1 with an historical account of the Project. This sets the scene, so to speak, by considering the professional and political events which led up to implementation.

Chapters 2 and 3 address the structure and content of the new curricula. In Chapter 2 the content of the new curricula is considered in terms of the knowledge component and how this guides practice and is in turn influenced by that practice. The importance of an integration of 'theory' and 'practice' is emphasised and the contribution of social sciences as the newest disciplines in an integrated curriculum is illustrated. Chapter 3 continues this latter theme by considering in detail the notion of 'integration' and how this is achieved through the inclusion of a sociology of nursing.

Chapters 4 and 5 deal with philosophical considerations. In Chapter 4 the nature of *care* as an existential concept is considered. The essential nature of caring in nursing is discussed and a rationale for incorporating care as the essential and fundamental core of the nursing curriculum is presented. Chapter

5 continues this philosophical theme by addressing the moral and ethical basis of nursing practice in the context of a managerial and technology-orientated health service. It proceeds to emphasise the importance of a moral and ethical consciousness in nursing and to illustrate how Ethics can be incorporated in the new curriculum.

Chapters 6 and 7 focus in on how learning experiences are organised in the new curricula. In Chapter 6 a transactional curriculum which is founded on negotiation between the three main bodies of 'actors' – students, teachers and clinicians – is advocated. The implications of a negotiated curriculum for each of the main actors, and the role changes which will be involved, are discussed. Chapter 7 continues this theme by considering the student experience, contrasting this with the pre-Project 2000 situation and addressing how students and indeed their teachers are growing and developing in their new roles.

In Chapters 8 and 9 the issues of managing change and resource management in the new curricula are addressed. Chapter 8 describes the process of radical change and the difficulties this presents. It goes on to provide a detailed account of one college's quest for validation, programme implementation and the linkage established between that college and a higher education institution. In Chapter 9 the management of resources as a vital element in Project 2000 implementation is analysed. The issues of resourcing innovation, library resources and student counselling services are given particular attention.

Chapter 10, the penultimate chapter, stresses the importance, even at this early stage, of addressing the important issues of course evaluation and review. It is emphasised that evaluation is a continuing and ongoing process. Particular attention is given to course organisation, theory and practice, student supervision, teaching and peer review and evaluation.

Chapter 11, the final chapter, is in essence a look to the future. The chapter takes as its vehicle the strategy for nursing of one of the four UK Health Departments, and considers how nursing and nurse education may control their own destinies by moving towards this future with courage and anticipation.

If our readers expect magical formulae in these chapters they will be sorely disappointed. What they will find instead is a reflection of themselves – the thoughts and ideas of educators like themselves who, just like themselves, are grappling with new problems and thinking about new solutions. Our hope, as the editors of this collection of papers, is that we have brought to our readers a number of the important issues in Project 2000 with an opportunity to see how some of our colleagues are addressing these. Our goal is that the papers will contribute to an ongoing debate, the outcome of which will be an advancement of the ideas, experiences and solutions presented in these chapters.

Mike Buckenham
Oliver Slevin
July 1992

Reference

United Kingdom Central Council for Nursing, Midwifery and Health Visiting. (1986). *Project 2000: A New Preparation for Practice,* London, UKCC

1

Education for the future: meeting changing needs

Janet James and David Jones

Introduction

This chapter describes how the profession arrived at its present position and the way Project 2000 has developed. It identifies the overall aims, policy influences and strategic directions and looks at how these are being carried forward to meet the health care needs of the 1990s. It concludes by commenting on the balance between political expediency and professional development.

Throughout history it has been necessary to change and develop the education and training of nurses, midwives and health visitors in order to meet the health care needs of society. The mid to late 1900s were marked by the recognition that minor alterations to curricula did not equip practitioners to cope with the rapidly changing content of health care. This acknowledgment of the need for radical change culminated in the Briggs report of 1972 which dominated discussion among the professions throughout the 1970s.

Its recommendations for a united profession, common portals of entry and continuing education throughout the practitioner's career were on the whole welcomed, but Government could not be persuaded to introduce the necessary legislation and funding partly because the professions were unable to demonstrate solidarity. However, in the late 1970s sufficient common ground was identified particularly in relation to the need to rationalise the provision of statutory and other registration, validation and accreditation systems and Government were convinced of the potential cost effectiveness of developing a new statutory framework.

The Nurses, Midwives and Health Visitors Act finally entered the statute book in May 1979. The Act established a United Kingdom Central Council for Nurses, Midwives and Health Visitors (UKCC) and four National Boards for Nursing, Midwifery and Health Visiting.

The UKCC was charged by the 1979 Act with regulation of the profession

Note
Throughout this chapter the word 'practitioner' is used as a generic term to describe a nurse, midwife or health visitor on any part of the professional register.

and specifically to 'maintain and improve standards of training and conduct'. Their task was therefore to resolve the conflicts.

> 'Going forward toward a unified profession which will enable all nurses, midwives and health visitors to benefit by what is good in each of its branches...bringing the whole of the wider professions up to the professional standards and individual accountability of the midwife (much of whose autonomy has in fact already been eroded by modern hospital practice); disseminating the ideal of preventive health care, which is the corner-stone of health visiting, throughout nursing; achieving a levelling up, rather than a levelling down, of practice and training.
> There are lessons to be learned from psychiatric nursing, sick children's nursing, district nursing, occupational health and so on, lessons about meeting the needs of the whole person rather than treating a disease in isolation.'
>
> Ross 1982

The creation of the new unified statutory structure was designed to decrease bureaucratic processes, prevent re-invention of the wheel and increase efficiency and economy of action. In addition and perhaps most importantly it could give greater political powers of negotiation by providing a body which would speak authoritatively on behalf of all members of the profession and which embodied within its remit the requirement for professional self regulation. However, between 1980 and 1983 there continued to be much inconclusive debate, uncertainty and dissatisfaction within the profession. This included concern at the existence of two levels of registered nurses.

In the summer of 1984 the UKCC established a project:

> 'to determine the education and training required for the professional practice of nursing, midwifery and health visiting in relation to the projected health care needs in the 1990s and beyond and to make recommendations.'

This became known as Project 2000. The Project group was constituted from the membership of the UKCC and was representative of the four countries of the UK and a wide variety of areas of professional practice.

From mid 1984 until early 1986 the UKCC sought to gauge the views of the professions before proposals for reform were put together. Project papers to clarify options were prepared, a video was made to stimulate discussions and to identify problems and a series of meetings was held throughout the UK. In May 1986 the UKCC published its major consultation report, *Project 2000: A New Preparation for Practice* (UKCC, 1986). This contained a detailed analysis of the case for change, described the different patterns of preparation in the four countries of the UK and outlined recommendations for change. Between May and the end of October 1986 the UKCC embarked upon a major exercise to consult nurses, midwives and health visitors and others about the proposals and the principles on which they were based.

The consultation was mainly a professional one but active opportunities were taken to brief health service chairmen, members and managers, representatives of the medical profession and other professional groups about the proposals and the thinking behind them in an attempt to secure their support.

In spite of their differences practitioners were drawn to the opportunity to raise the credibility of education and training towards the development of 'a knowledgeable doer', but each discipline wished to preserve its individual skills and autonomy within the general move towards reform. Many other professional groups within the NHS were less enthusiastic about proposals which plainly sought to increase the professional status of practitioners. These initially exerted pressure on the Government to resist the proposals but eventually had to concede the need for change if health care was to continue to develop and improve.

The UKCC engaged the management consultancy firm Price Waterhouse to examine the cost and manpower implications of their proposals and the issues involved in implementing changes on the scales envisaged. By November 1986 the results of consultation with the professions had been fully analysed and a strategy for educational reform was developed and agreed. Price Waterhouse produced *Project Paper 8* (Price Waterhouse, 1988). This included a cost benefit analysis of the proposals which the Government found persuasive. Even though they were not convinced that the workforce targets identified were achievable it was evident that existing training was too wasteful to continue and that a new strategy was needed. At its meeting in January 1987 the UKCC agreed its policy on education and training reform and this was presented to the Ministers of the four health departments of the UK on 5th February 1987. It was significant that the Project 2000 proposals had. been presented by the UKCC but were put forward as a five-body document. The full support of the four national boards was achieved after the publication of the Report.

In retrospect it is apparent that Government approval was granted because Project 2000 offered the opportunity to prepare the professions to work within changes brought about by the reforms of the NHS and the general education system. Although this should have been apparent to nurse leaders at the time it is suggested that reality is only just beginning to dawn on the majority of practitioners involved in implementing Project 2000. The provision of a practitioner able to function at diploma level, that is to understand and apply theories to problematic situations, critically evaluate their usefulness and produce creative solutions is entirely consistent with the need to have a well trained, flexible human resource which can be deployed to work in any care situation, hospital or community, thus making maximum use of a decreasing level of resources in the most efficient and cost-effective way and where possible without expensive re-training. In May 1988 the Secretary of State, John Moore, accepted the Project 2000 proposals subject to: further work being carried out on widening the entry gate; the professions supporting the development of the support worker role; provision of opportunities for enrolled nurses to progress to first level registration; and further exploration of the role of the specialist practitioner.

In October 1988 Len Peach, Chief Executive of the English NHS Management Board, advised general managers that it was necessary to create a framework and infrastructure for change by identifying schools of nursing which might begin Project 2000 training and to draw up implementation plans so that one school from each region should move to a Project 2000 basis by autumn 1989. These schools were to become the demonstration districts leading the way in the new initiative and advising their colleagues and other health authorities who were to follow.

The aim of Project 2000

The UKCC Chairperson, Audrey Emerton gave a clear statement in 1988 on the aim of Project 2000:

'The health care services in the UK are approaching a major crisis and urgent action is needed not simply to solve short term problems but to lay the foundations for more sound education and personnel policies. Prospects are bleak and imaginative action is needed if we are to avoid the further erosion of standards and the use of unqualified staff and students to undertake work for which they have neither the experience nor the training. Many nurses, midwives and health visitors would like even more radical changes but the strategy will:
- provide the necessary levels and types of nursing for the future and which Government plans and health authorities' strategies demand;
- reflect the principal aspirations of the professions to provide better care;
- in the medium term prove to be more cost effective;
- maintain the pre-eminent position of British nursing in the world;
- address issues of finance and manpower realistically.

These proposals are not intended simply to enhance the professions. In embarking upon this exercise the UKCC took as its starting point the health care needs of society. These remain our principal concern and I believe that patients and clients above all will stand to benefit from our proposals for change.'

The policy background

There were three important factors which underpinned the need for change. These were:
- demographic changes – a significant decrease in the number of young people available for recruitment to the health care professions;
- the Government's sustained emphasis on cost effectiveness and value for money within health care;
- Government policy which emphasises the prevention of ill health and provision of health care within the community.

It is obvious that reforms in nursing do not occur within a vacuum; they are set within a wider political context. Project 2000 implied not merely a new pre-registration curriculum but a pervasive influence on every aspect of the nursing service. It was, however, only one change among the multitude that the NHS had to deal with in the late 1980s and early 1990s, including clinical regrading, quality assurance programmes, rationalisation and restructuring of services, the introduction of internal markets and new relationships between purchasers and providers of services and education.

Some of these changes were evident in the Government White Paper, *Putting Patients First* (1979) published before Project 2000 was developed, whilst others would emerge during Project 2000's implementation. These include the reforms described in *Working for Patients* (1989) and in particular its *Education and Training Working Paper 10* (1989) and *Caring for People – Community Care in the Next Decade and Beyond* (1990).

The task of the profession's leaders was to anticipate which changes would have maximum impact and prepare a project which would on the one hand enable practitioners to deal with the changes and on the other meet the Government's requirements for the future, without sacrificing professional principles, skills or identities. The latter was vital in order to secure the approval and funding necessary for the implementation of major change.

With this in mind the UKCC agreed four broad criteria to assess the options for change against, these were:

'the effect on standards of care at present and in the future particularly in relation to health promotion and prevention of disease as well as care of the sick;
an increase in job satisfaction so as to reduce wastage and attract new recruits through improvements and standards of care;
realistic costs and manpower effects and consideration of practical issues of implementation;
any changes should improve standards of training in accordance with the 1979 Act and that proposals should reflect the profession's concerns.'

UKCC 1987

After much debate the UKCC produced a strategy with two inter-linked elements; these were education and training reforms, and proposals to improve manpower supply and retention.

Education and training reforms

Plans for the future were centred on the creation of a single level of practitioner, more enquiring, able to gather information and make an assessment of need, devise a plan of care, and implement, monitor and evaluate it. The new practitioner was to be actively involved in the delivery of care, not simply a supervisor of it, and upon registration would be able to work in non-institutional or institutional settings.

The phrase 'knowledgeable doer' was coined to sum up the new practitioner: a person educated to diploma or degree level with transferable intellectual and clinical skills, able to provide a personalised health care service as well as to cope with the welter of new tasks emerging such as analysing skill mixes, setting standards of care, taking part in audits and quality assurance programmes and local budget management. The new practitioner must develop the confidence and assertiveness to survive and flourish in a constantly changing environment. In order to achieve these ambitious aims new pre-registration programmes were designed to facilitate the development of higher order cognitive skills. These were to consist of a common foundation programme and branch programmes

15

designed to reduce the amount of overlap and repetition between different disciplines and between some of the pre- and post-registration trainings.

There has been disagreement among the professional groups on the benefit of core professional themes within common foundation programmes. Some authors (Telford, 1985 and Allen, 1992) observe that the smaller speciality groups may find their own skills diluted by a conformity to the ideals, values and preoccupations of the dominant branch. These concerns will need to be addressed in future so that opportunities are not lost for shared learning in which all contributions are recognised as having a unique value. In similar vein concerns have been expressed that supernumerary status and the move towards higher education have the potential to increase the theory/practice gap.

The National Foundation for Educational Research (NFER) is conducting a longitudinal study of the implementation of these new pre-registration courses. One of their interim reports (Payne et al. 1991) shows that some teachers believe the courses might not provide nurses with the experience needed to develop clinical skills, whilst others express a relief that students no longer have to repeat nursing procedures again and again with questionable benefit. Both students and educationalists have expressed some initial difficulty in maximising the potential of supernumerary status, and have yet to evaluate the change which will occur towards the end of the courses when students begin to provide a 20 per cent service contribution.

The issues surrounding the replacement of a student workforce on the wards (such as the adequacy of the level of replacement and the skill mix within different schemes, the cost and complexity of health care assistant training and the impact on existing staff) remain the day to day concerns of service managers. In many respects the formulae on which funding bids were calculated by demonstration districts were based on unknown variables and need to be reviewed in the light of experience as does the mechanism within the health authorities for directing funding to these areas. Jowett et al. (1991) state:

'the centrality of educationalists carrying service staff with them and bringing about Project 2000 changes – so that there is truly an education/service partnership – has been repeatedly emphasised, as has the constant and continuing input of time and effort which will be needed to achieve that partnership ... but there is also awareness of and concern about, the ever-increasing demands on service staff (and the impact of these on their morale) resulting from all the current educational and management changes – as well as changing care patterns. The success of Project 2000 may depend upon the support which they receive as much as on the support they give to students.'

The need to develop links with higher education institutions has coincided with major changes in the structuring and function of general education provision. Jowett et al. (1991) note that serious financial difficulties and worsening staff ratios in some institutions now dependent for growth and survival on attracting an increasing number of students, cannot but affect attitudes to the developing links with colleges of nursing and midwifery. In many cases a measure of self-defensiveness and suspicion between teachers and lecturers as well as between the different institutions has had to be overcome before the agreements necessary and beneficial to both could be reached. The level of participation and collaboration between colleges of nursing and institutes of higher education varies considerably among the demonstration districts but all must move towards a better understanding if the potential benefits are to be maximised.

One significant problem is the confusion which exists on both sides over what diploma level study actually constitutes. This is compounded by the apparent tensions between acceptable levels of pure and applied theoretical study and the difficulty of convincing colleagues in higher education that time spent in the practical areas is spent applying theories into practice and not just performing routine tasks. There is a need to resolve precisely what higher education should contribute to the courses and to bring together the various elements into a coherent, well integrated whole and then relate the level of work and its contents to students' past experience and educational attainment.

Some positive changes have already occurred. For example, joint professional and academic validation of courses has been achieved despite the difficulties outlined above and, to the credit of all concerned, the mystique surrounding higher education has been dispelled for many teachers. However, this tends to include only those who are at the centre of the changes and there is a need to extend the range of human contact out to those peripherally involved.

The development of academic credit accumulation and transfer schemes has provided an opportunity at last for the professions to establish the academic currency of existing courses and will provide a helpful basis for planning and developing the new framework for continuing professional education and training (ENB, 1990). The next challenge is to devise a means of accrediting professional as well as academic development so that the framework can support and integrate the practitioner's progress in both dimensions. As the professions are rooted in practice and the prime aim of reform is to meet changing health care needs, it is vital that this opportunity to structure future professional development is used to bring theory and practice closer together and to close rather than extend the existing theory/practice gap.

Project 2000 identified the need to develop a 'specialist practitioner' role. This would be based in either hospital or community and involve specialist knowledge in either health promotion, specific diseases or disorders and nursing interventions. Some roles would combine teaching with practice and some would be team leader roles. All would have completed additional education and training programmes. This recognition of the value of clinical expertise was welcomed as long overdue. Many practitioners believed that the traditional routes for progression into education or management provided narrow fields of opportunity and a decreasing number of posts as services were rationalised. The specialist practitioner offered an attractive alternative, though it remains to be seen whether the development of clinical expertise will be appropriately rewarded in the grading structure.

Existing post-registration education varies in both quality and quantity depending on the level of funding local health authorities have been prepared to invest in it, and on the interest and motivation of education and service providers. With the development of pre-registration education well underway the UKCC turned its attention to the statutory and mandatory changes which would regulate post-registration education and improve standards. These included the development of a 'live' register, a requirement to demonstrate professional updating before re-registration and compulsory return to practice programmes for those absent for more than five years.

In many centres work has already begun to rationalise post-registration programmes and to assess and accredit their academic value. Common core curricula are developing for both hospital and community courses emphasising the value of shared learning between different disciplines in nursing and in some cases with other professional groups, such as social workers, but maintaining specialist components for the development of specific knowledge, skills and attitudes.

The National Boards recognise that development opportunities are limited for many nurses and have been working towards a more coherent approach which would give all practitioners the opportunity of a clearly defined and well planned programme of professional development. In 1990 the ENB published its framework for continuing professional education and training and in 1991 began to consider guidelines for establishing consortia with higher education. In 1991 the UKCC provided the details of its Post Registration Education and Practice Project (PREPP) which describes the stages of induction, primary practice, advanced practice and consultancy for registered nurses in their professional development.

The enrolled nurses have been both winners and losers in the Project 2000 evolutionary process. Many felt devalued by the negative discussions of their role and the cessation of training (by default) which came early in the Project 2000 changes. There was no doubt their choice of job opportunities would be limited as their numbers steadily decreased in the workplace but their contribution is of great value and in many instances enrolled nurses form the backbone of a stable and reliable nursing service. Education and service managers have a responsibility to provide relevant and appropriate opportunities for professional development for this essential group within the new frameworks for continuing education.

After a slow start there has been an increase in opportunities for enrolled nurses to convert from second to first level nurse, either through a conversion course or where appropriate by taking additional attempts at first level examinations. The development of new open learning programmes which are flexible in length and in content has not only increased the number of places available to enrolled nurses but has pushed back the boundaries of educational development and adult models of learning in nursing. In the past nurses have been criticised for their inflexibility and tendency to take a rule-following attitude rather than being prepared to develop analytical and problem-solving skills. This tendency was reinforced through rigid education and training practices. The new pre- and post-registration and conversion programmes attempt to overcome this problem and are designed to develop a more reflective practitioner.

The principles of flexible training are extending into the preparation of health care assistants. When the health care assistant was first proposed practitioners were convinced that they should be involved in defining the role and that local health authorities should provide competency-based training in line with a nationally produced accreditation package. However, there were considerable delays in the arrival of national guidelines and many health authorities began to develop their own schemes based on information provided by the National Health Service Training Authority (NHSTA — now the NHS Training Directorate or NHSTD). It is evident that nurses should direct the development of the health care assistant role and be involved in supervising and assessing individual achievement of competencies if they are to maintain their control over the standards of care.

In line with the original Project 2000 recommendations there have been improvements in the education and training environment. The recommendations that teachers should be qualified at degree level has been endorsed and local strategies have developed for achieving that goal. On the whole teachers have been aware of their need to develop academic skills and have willingly entered into this area of professional development. This has enhanced the credibility of colleges of nursing and midwifery with institutes of higher education and given the teachers a wider and deeper range of experience and knowledge to offer their students. There are, however, still pockets of resistance to supporting teachers with adequate funding and study leave, but these issues will have to be addressed if institutions are to gain academic approval. In addition there are new pressures on teachers to enhance their clinical liaison and personal tutor roles as well as to prepare, teach and mark a still unfamiliar diploma level course which involves a greater degree of subject specialisation. The phasing out of clinical teachers and the move toward a single grade of nurse teacher has been another factor in the process of change. The need to cope with all these pressures and anxieties cannot be over-estimated in the current climate and course leaders have a key role in supporting their teaching teams and helping them through the present situation.

Many clinical practitioners find themselves under similar pressure at the moment as they seek to upgrade their knowledge and skills in order to provide a stimulating and supportive environment for students in placements and to demonstrate a high standard of professional practice. Evidence of their considerable achievements in this area is provided through the clinical audits.

Human resources in education and service have been overstretched by the rapid introduction of Project 2000 which gave little time for adaptation to new roles, structures and functions. Though the NFER note a continuing commitment on both sides to make the changes work they comment that the number of students involved places considerable demands on physical and human resources and militates against the student-centred approaches which are crucial in the new courses. The necessity for formal lectures to such large groups and the difficulties in taking account of individual students' past experiences and education when arranging and supervising placements are obvious manifestations. Similarly, what could be seen as a transitional deficiency, the lack of adequate library resources, appears to be a much longer term issue. The important lesson here is that large groups and core themes are only cost effective up to a certain point and when the quality of the students' learning and experience is compromised beyond the teachers' abilities to solve the problems their role is to protect the student interests and not the throughput of cannon fodder. Otherwise there is no advantage in providing supernumerary status and a revolutionary new course. On a similar theme there has been a huge effort to provide 'top up' training and preparation for clinical staff who will guide the students in practice settings. If not managed carefully this important work can become an endless treadmill for the teachers responsible as more and more placements, institutional and non-institutional, have to be brought on stream and there is a constant need to keep up with staff turnover in areas which have been previously prepared.

Manpower supply and retention

When the Project 2000 proposals were put forward they were designed in part to alleviate the serious manpower problems which faced the NHS. Demographic changes showed a severe downturn in young people available for the labour market, and although the problem was not evenly spread throughout the UK, severe and sustained problems were predicted in some areas. The decline was predicted to reach its lowest point by 1995. *Project Paper 8* (UKCC, 1987) gives a detailed breakdown of the problem.

The UKCC originally estimated that about 32,000 students would need to enter educational programmes in 1995 to guarantee the full implementation of its proposals. Demographic projections suggested the likely supply of entrants assuming no other policy changes were made would be 16,000 producing a shortfall of 16,000. Two solutions were proposed: a reduction in the demand for new entrants and an increase in the supply of trainees.

Reducing the demand for new entrants depended on reducing the wastage of qualified staff, reducing educational wastage and increasing the number of 'returners'. The UKCC proposed that the NHS management should define and set new objectives for improving the retention of qualified staff. There were at the time both national (Price Waterhouse, 1988) and local (Hart 1989) studies which identified reasons for wastage and potential solutions, but as yet nurses at grass roots level have experienced little practical change in their working environment or practices to alleviate the problems.

The drive towards increased efficiency and economy and the new contractual relationships between the purchasers and providers of professional education are leading to the development of more sophisticated management information systems and a clearer picture of wastage and turnover. But to an extent efforts to analyse and act on this information have been overtaken by events as managers and practitioners struggle to implement other aspects of the Government reforms. Although some of these may have raised stress levels and dissatisfaction among nurses they have not substantially increased wastage because they are counter-balanced by a downturn in the general economic climate and a high level of general unemployment. In the meantime it is hoped that providing a better pre-registration training and greater opportunities for post-registration professional development will contribute to practitioners feeling valued and enable them to see a long term route to career development.

It is as yet too early to determine whether the Project 2000 programmes have achieved the objective of reducing attrition rates during training. However, it is expected that supernumerary status will reduce stress levels for students particularly during their early practice placements and there is some anecdotal evidence that wastage in the first two years of the programme has been reduced.

Further studies are required to demonstrate whether there are additional factors associated with teaching styles and educational methods which may have both positive and negative effects on student attrition. For example, widening the entry gate may result in some students not completing the more demanding diploma level programmes.

The UKCC suggest that the number of 'returners' to nursing could be increased by improved advertising and re-orientation programmes, more flexible working arrangements and greater provision of support facilities for those with family commitments. Most practitioners welcome the fact that re-orientation programmes are now a statutory requirement for those absent for more than five years but a serious question hangs over who will pay for the privilege of re-orientation programmes, the employer or the nurse who wishes to return to the labour market. The answer is probably that it could be either, depending on service requirements.

The issues of flexible working arrangements and greater provision of support facilities have been largely ignored. This is disappointing in a profession which has a predominantly female workforce and is very familiar with the difficulties associated with balancing a commitment to work and caring for dependants. These problems are not new; they have been identified and discussed time and again since the inception of the NHS and yet the professions seem unable to move from rigid traditional work patterns and remain the prisoners of history. This is not simply a problem which affects the service sector. Colleges of nursing have been very slow in introducing part time or flexible working hours and job share schemes for their staff and even slower to offer part time and flexible courses for students. Perhaps the current emphasis on consumer-led education will help to force these changes through. The flexible conversion programmes can give a lead here. They are designed to meet the needs of students by allowing them to decide whether to study part or full time and by using open learning to offer a choice of study content, pace, place and time.

In all the areas discussed above there is an increasing acknowledgment of the contribution made by practitioners within the independent sector and of the need to include them in the processes of education reform and manpower planning. The early work in this area shows mutual benefit for both public and private sector participants. For example, private sector placements are being audited as suitable areas for the new pre-registration programmes and conversion courses. This widens the scope of practical experience available to students and offers them an alternative view of health care. At the same time the professional development opportunities for staff within those areas are increasing as, for example, enrolled nurses come forward for conversion courses and health care assistants for National Council for Vocational Qualifications (NCVQ) accreditation. Traditional barriers to communication are breaking down and the two types of service provision are beginning to learn from each other. These lessons will ultimately benefit the standard of patient care in both areas.

A number of measures were originally proposed to increase the supply of entrants to education programmes. These included increasing the number of male entrants and mature students and widening the entry gate to training. The number of male entrants is gradually increasing as is the number of mature students. There are a number of possible reasons for these changes, some connected to the provision of a more attractive pre-registration training and a higher academic standard, some to the widening entry gate which now ranges through access courses, DC tests, formal qualifications and in future could include NCVQs and other types of accreditation of previous learning activities. Undoubtedly an unexpected influence has been the high level of unemployment and reduced job opportunities in other spheres.

The costs and benefits considered

The UKCC's original argument was that the cost of the innovations described above would be balanced by the rationalisation of the total pattern of education and training, the enhanced lifetime participation of qualified staff in the workforce and their increased productivity.

There certainly has been a concerted effort at rationalisation. Groups of schools have amalgamated into colleges, and groups of courses have amalgamated into core courses with specialist branches or modules. There is evidence that cost savings will occur in the future but these are not clearly available yet as most centres are continuing at their previous level of funding during the initial setting up period and some have received pump priming money to help them on their way. However, many would argue that their level of productivity has increased while resources, human and material, have remained constant or decreased through an increased level of staff taking early retirement. One thing is clear: much more attention is being paid to financial management and income generation than ever before and there will be increasing pressure from the Government and the regional health authorities to demonstrate economies, efficiency and effectiveness in education and service management. The professions will need to demonstrate their ability to evaluate their own practices and review performance at every level, and to define and advocate a high quality of education and service if standards of health care are to be maintained and improved. Whether or not there is enhanced lifetime participation or increased productivity on the part of a more effectively prepared workforce remains to be seen, but there is already and will continue to be a great deal of research interest in this area.

Conclusion

The Project 2000 proposals were designed to enable members of the profession to make a greater contribution to the planning, assessment and delivery of services in a climate of austerity rather than expansion. The UKCC recognised that all professionals were going to have to fight harder to ensure they had the resources to meet existing and future health and social care needs.

Project Paper 6 (UKCC 1985) noted that from the point of registration future practitioners would need to understand the planning process, information systems and policy debates which surround their work. They would need to evaluate their own practice, argue the case for particular services and defend them against criticism. This entailed analysing local and national health information, using limited resources efficiently and contributing to continuous audit of health services as well as identifying health care needs. Assessment of community as well as individual client needs would be part of a re-orientation towards providing care in the community.

None of these suggestions were entirely new but Project 2000 sought to bring them together through a process of re-orientation which implied change at every level from creating new relationships with clients through new ways of thinking about teaching and learning, new pre- and post-registration education programmes and a new pattern of regulation and support by the statutory bodies. If this were to be a success the first requirements were a united vision of what the professions could achieve and how this relates and responds to health care needs. How far the profession has been successful in achieving unity of vision is debatable. There has been a wealth of opportunities for practitioners, managers and teachers from all the different disciplines to discuss their ideas and concerns and in many cases to work out mutually beneficial solutions. However, much remains to be done in this area: many of the old disagreements and divisions persist and the smaller professional groups continue to feel marginalised and therefore devalued in the process of change. Sensitivity to this issue and a willingness to understand the needs, perspectives and contributions of all members of the profession is required at every level from national and local policy making and implementation through to interpersonal relationships among colleagues working together.

As to the potential for improving relationships between education and service colleagues, in large measure this has been the concern of individual colleges and their host health authorities who recognise the purpose of co-operation as combining the expertise of all parties to their mutual benefit in the development of relevant and appropriate curricula which seek to reduce the theory/practice gap and improve the quality of care. It can also prevent impractical or unrealistic planning and secure the service support necessary for successful implementation of new programmes (James and Marr, 1992).

The difference in levels of collaboration has varied depending on the motivation of key individuals and their managers. The task for the future is to maintain and improve those relationships through the difficulties of working out purchaser and provider relationships and new contractual arrangements. For nurse teachers the background to these changes has been complicated by the rationalisation of schools of nursing and midwifery into large colleges. This may be a difficult process but it is also one which can lead to a greater sharing of ideas and a levelling up rather than a levelling down of educational standards in which students gain the benefit of a wider pool of skills and expertise.

Despite the uncertainty of working through the Project 2000 changes, the large workloads and the stress of meeting deadlines, the NFER studies suggest that people have valued their experience of involvement in Project 2000. Many were keen to develop the process of consultation and team work and felt their involvement led to personal and professional development. A firm commitment is evident to the changes even though there are still widespread reservations about the type of nurse Project 2000 will produce, how easily they will fit into the traditional culture of the NHS and what sort of employment will be available for them. It is too early to measure the outcomes and their effect on health care yet but research has been commissioned to that end. In the present value-for-money culture both the Government and the statutory bodies will await the results with interest.

Dame Audrey Emerton chose her words carefully when she stated that

Project 2000 was not intended simply to enhance the professions and that the health care needs of society remained a principal concern so that patients and clients should benefit from the proposals for change. It is important to keep this focus in mind as Project 2000 is carried forward into the 1990s because it is the justification for change and it was the argument which persuaded the Government to approve and fund the proposals.

In bringing about such major reforms there were compromises to be achieved between political expediency, social conscience and professional interests. It was understood that preparing the professions to become a flexible and responsive workforce capable of surviving in a turbulent environment would meet the Government's requirement for NHS reforms, but this had to be achieved in a way which would protect the best interests of the different client groups and which would maintain and improve standards of care. Raising the credibility of nursing and the status of the profession was seen by many outsiders as a by-product of the change (and in some cases an unpopular one) which could aid recruitment and retention. The more astute within the profession may have played its importance down initially but recognised that if nurses were to gain and use political power to influence the delivery of care this could only be achieved by raising the status of the profession so that it was respected as an equal voice in the health care debate of the future.

The 1990s will be as challenging a decade as the 1980s were. The education reforms proposed in Project 2000 have really only just begun and there is as much to do in carrying them forward as has already been achieved in the implementation of new pre-registration and conversion programmes.

References

Allen, C. (1992). Foundation for success, *Nursing Times* , Vol 88 No. 2.

Briggs, A. (1972). *A Report of the Committee on Nursing* , London, HMSO.

Emerton, A. (1987). *Project 2000 – Government Approval in Principle*, UKCC.

ENB. (1990). *Framework for Continuing Professional Education & Training for Nurses, Midwives & Health Visitors, Project Paper 3*, London, ENB.

Government White Paper. (1979). *Putting Patients First,* London, HMSO.

Government White Paper. (1989). *Working for Patients,* London, HMSO.

Government White Paper. (1989). *Education & Training, Working Paper 10 of Working for Patients,* London, HMSO.

Government White Paper. (1990). *Caring for People: Community Care the Next Decade & Beyond,* London, HMSO.

Hart, E. (1989). A qualitative study of factors affecting retention & turnover amongst nursing staff in paediatrics & care of the elderly research report for Trent Regional Health Authority.

James, J. and Marr, J. (1992). *Development and Validation of an Open Learning Second to First Level Nurse Education Course,* London, ENB.

Jowett, S. Walton, I. and Payne, S. (1991). *The NFER Project 2000 Research – An Introduction and some Interim Issuess, Project Paper 2,* Slough, NFER.

Payne, S., Jowett, S. and Walton, I. (1991). *Nurse Teachers in Project 2000 The Experience of Planning and Initial Implementation , Project Paper 3,* Slough, NFER.

Price Waterhouse. (1988). *Nurse Retention & Recruitment , A Matter of Priority* , Regional Health Boards and Authorities in England, Scotland and Wales.

Ross, T. (1982). Election special supplement,. *Nursing Mirror* , 20 Oct 1982.

Telford, A. (1985). Interpersonal skills training: therapeutic tool and professional necessity, *Community Psychiatric Nursing Journal,* Vol 5 No. 3.

UKCC. (1985). *Project 2000: Introducing Project 2000, Project Paper 1,* London, UKCC.
UKCC. (1985). *Project 2000: Facing the Future, Project Paper 6,* London, UKCC.
UKCC. (1986). *Project 2000: A New Preparation for Practice,* London, UKCC.
UKCC. (1987). *Project 2000: Counting the Cost, Project Paper 8,* London, UKCC.
UKCC. (1987). *Project 2000: The Final Proposals,Project Paper 9,* London, UKCC.
UKCC. (1990). *Report of the Post Registration Education and Practice Project,* London, UKCC.

2

Knowledgeable doing:
the theoretical basis for practice

Oliver Slevin

Education is not acquiring a stock of ready-made ideas, images, sentiments, beliefs and so forth; it is learning to look, to listen, to think, to feel, to imagine, to believe, to understand, to choose and to wish.

Michael Oakeshott, 1989

Introduction

Implementation of Project 2000 commenced in the United Kingdom in late 1989/early 1990 with the very first courses in thirteen Demonstration Districts in England. It was intended that these first programmes would serve as models or sources of information for subsequent waves of nurse education institutions implementing the Project. Research being carried out under the auspices of the National Foundation for Educational Research has already resulted in useful interim reports on progress within the first Demonstration Districts (see: Leonard and Jowett, 1990; Jowett et al. 1991; Payne et al. 1991). In Scotland and Wales progressive implementation approaches have been adopted, while in Northern Ireland a 'big bang' strategy was chosen – with all Colleges of Nursing commencing Project 2000 programmes between October 1990 and Spring 1991.

As we move forward with implementation of the Project, ward staff and students – the new Project 2000 students – have been heard to say some interesting things. Some ward staff have been asking how these students will ever become competent nurses if they just come to the wards to observe and do not work. One actually asked the author if it would be alright for the students to help with making the beds and bathing the patients. Some students have been expressing anxiety about not being able to get involved in 'actual nursing', which was what they commenced the course to do! After several weeks on the course, during which time they had been on observational community placements, they were becoming intensely concerned about the lack of opportunity to 'do' nursing, as they understood it i.e. doing injections, dressing wounds etc.

Now we must, to some extent, keep such comments in perspective. Project 2000 is a major innovation. And even those who are still not fully acquainted with its detail are at least becoming conscious that nursing is facing significant structural and functional change. It is in the nature of human beings that, in periods of rapid and major change, rumours and misinterpretations spread like a plague. Even the most effective communication networks, orientation programmes and change agents do not completely prevent the most outlandish interpretations on the 'shop-floor'.

Irrespective of the apparent lack of a sound basis for rumours we should never, if we are wise, ignore them. In the case of Project 2000, the commitment to practice and direct nursing care is fundamental. Even the title of the original Project report (UKCC, 1986) emphasises this commitment. Project 2000 was entitled, A New *Preparation* for *Practice* (author's italics). The Project represents a *new* and *better* education to inform the practice of nursing. Much of the rumour seems to be based on the erroneous idea that:

Being more academic and more educationally advanced means being less practical and less able or competent.

This view must be dispelled, as must any risk that it should become a reality. An essential premise in Project 2000 is that:

The new educational programme will provide a sound body of knowledge which informs and enhances practice.

Knowledge is therefore not antithetical to good practice; rather, good practice is *dependent* on sound, up-to-date knowledge. It is this issue which this paper addresses. It is argued that a broad knowledge base is essential, that this knowledge must be integrated with nursing in a systematic way and that, within this broad approach, the social sciences have a valuable contribution to make.

Informed practice

A simplified view of how nursing has developed in the UK in recent years is presented in Figure 1. Prior to the mid-1980s, the apprenticeship structure in nurse education was directed toward a procedure and task-oriented approach to practice. Nurses were rule-orientated and were not encouraged – indeed were discouraged – in regard to reflecting upon or questioning practice. They were 'doers' and not 'thinkers'. Practice was essentially tradition-driven and based on a medical model of diagnosis – treatment/care – cure – discharge. Even in psychiatric nursing, where a more holistic and interpersonal model of nursing might have been expected, Powell (1982) found students were actively discouraged from developing personal relationships with their patients.

Questions are begged here as to why we adopted this almost mindless doing in our professional practice. A number of explanations may be suggested. For example, Menzies (1960) has suggested that this impersonal, task orientated approach reflected the use of *social* defence mechanisms in nursing, i.e., the approach avoided close personal relationships with patients and the risk of the stress and trauma this might involve. Doing something with *things*, concentrating on procedures rather than interpersonal processes, was much easier. This tendency may indeed have extended into our educational endeavours. Schon (1987) draws attention to the tendency – in both professional practice and professional education – to concentrate on the technical, the scientific, the instrumental,

Figure 1 A temporal progression

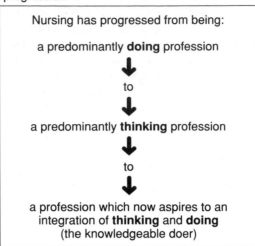

```
Nursing has progressed from being:

a predominantly doing profession
              ↓
             to
              ↓
a predominantly thinking profession
              ↓
             to
              ↓
a profession which now aspires to an
integration of thinking and doing
     (the knowledgeable doer)
```

rather than the more complex issues professionals face in their day to day work. Thus, in an activity such as nurse education, it is easier to 'teach' life sciences, technical procedures and rules for practice than to come to grips with fundamentally more complex human issues such as the nature of caring relationships and the business of living and working within them. Others, subscribing to a consensus view of society, suggest that a social order explanation provides insight. That is, nurses were socialised into behaving in this way to maintain the power structures in illness-orientated medical care. However, a third explanation would lay the blame to some extent at our own door. We simply may not have educated ourselves to be more thinking, reflective, risk-taking practitioners; we may have chosen to passively follow tradition, to do things in certain ways simply because that is how we always did them.

The introduction of new curricula, particularly in England and Northern Ireland, in the early to mid-1980s represented a change in direction. In Northern Ireland these new curricula were essentially role-based in that they:

(a)   addressed the role of the nurse in the clinical situation, and

(b)   identified the knowledge and skills elements to be addressed in preparing for this role.

A typical example was the *Syllabus for Part 5 of the Register – Mental Handicap Nursing* (NBNI, 1985) which identified the following role elements:

(i)   a set of competencies or skill-related capacities;

(ii)   a code of professional conduct, as laid down by the UKCC (1984);

(iii) a model for caring for mentally-handicapped people, which encompassed education and training, normalisation and individual rights and obligations as well as personal care.

The 'new' curricula, as they were referred to, emphasised a problem-centred approach to planned, individualised care – the nursing process method. There was a significant up-dating of the knowledge base, particularly as regards the social, behavioural and communication sciences.

The problem was that, by the mid-1980s, a pattern of disengagement from practice seemed to have developed. The best educated nurses i.e. first level practitioners, were those who were least involved in direct care. There was a tendency for first level nurses to be more involved in administrative duties, in planning care and in directing it 'at arms-length'. Most direct care was being provided by enrolled or second level nurses, students, and auxiliaries. Indeed, the more educated and experienced first level nurses became, the more they tended to move into non-direct care activities such as management and teaching. Organisational structures and grading/remunerative arrangements served only to augment this drift away from direct care. Nurses i.e. first level nurses, were increasingly becoming *thinkers* rather than *doers*.

The philosophy underlying Project 2000 is essentially an attempt to reverse this drift. The idea is that a new, single level of practitioner – supported by an *assistant* and with access to the leadership, guidance and advice of an *advanced practitioner* – will be primarily concerned with care delivery. Nurses will be provided with a high quality education directed specifically at a more informed practice. Nurses will be directly involved in practice. This practice will be health as well as illness or disability orientated. The new practitioner will be capable of problem-solving and sound practice in rapidly-changing situations, and be capable of functioning at a level of competence in both institutional and non-institutional situations. *Thinking* and *doing* would now be brought together in the new concept of the *knowledgeable doer*.

The knowledge which underpins practice

This integration of knowledge and practice begs a fundamental question as to what knowledge is valid in this context. That is, what knowledge is essential for informing practice. Henderson (1990) states that:

> 'The keynote to Project 2000 – is total care based on sound knowledge of

Biophysiology	Psychology	Sociology	Ecology
(the body)	(the mind)	(relationships with other people)	(relationships with the planet)'

There are problems with this statement, particularly if it is interpreted (as indeed it only can be!) as being a comprehensive taxonomy of the knowledge base of nursing. The most fundamental problem is perhaps that it is all about 'ologies'. That is, it is a knowledge base which is exclusively scientific in its orientation. This bias toward the scientific is slightly worrying. It is to an extent reflected in the recently published strategy statements on nursing in the UK, such as *A Strategy for Nursing* (Department of Health, 1989) and *A Strategy for Nursing, Midwifery and Health Visiting in Northern Ireland* (DHSS, 1991). The latter strategy statement strongly advocates the need to base nursing on sound research evidence. One cannot of course argue with this. This new Strategy is both courageous and laudable in its commitment where it states that:

> 'Nurses will use an analytic research-based approach in identifying, intervening and evaluating health issues', (and)

'Nurses must be able to undertake or be involved in research, to interpret and evaluate research findings and apply these where appropriate.'

This view is widely held in nursing. For example, Hockey (1987) states that:

'Legally, a professional nurse in the UK is held responsible for his or her actions and has to be able to defend them on the basis of the latest knowledge. The latest available knowledge must be based on research because this is the only way by which the body of knowledge can be changed or extended.'

However, if we accept the sciences as being dominant in nursing, if we view research as 'the scientific method' and as such the sole source of valid nursing knowledge, there is a risk of narrowing and de-humanising our professional base. The vital importance of research-derived scientific knowledge is not being disvalued here. Rather it is argued that the concept of knowledgeable doer must have a broader knowledge base. As indicated in Figure 2, the premise is that nursing must be informed by different kinds of knowledge. That is, not only the sciences, but the study of logic and the humanities. In essence the life sciences, social sciences etc. and 'logic' give us a science of nursing; the humanities and skills acquisition – ranging from the level of novice to what Benner (1984) described as the level of intuitive expertise or excellence – lead us to an art of nursing. However, such conceptual frameworks reflect a tidiness and compartmentalisation which does not exist in reality. Indeed some would argue with the classification suggested in Figure 2. Is politics an art or science form? Does logic correctly reside to the science side of this schema, and is reflection a process of logic, a humanistic endeavour or a professional skill? For the purpose of the point being made here, these questions matter little. Nursing – art *and* science – is about an integration of *all* relevant knowledge to inform practice.

It should also be recognised that the idea of knowledge informing practice can suggest an exclusively linear relationship. In scientific terminology, this takes the form of 'theory-testing' which is a common positivistic scientific approach. That is, a theory is posited and then tested through scientific enquiry – usually of an experimental nature – in a top-down way (Merton, 1968). When established as 'proven', the knowledge is applied to practice.

There are essentially two problems in adopting this narrow perspective. Firstly, a theory-testing or top-down approach imposes knowledge on the nursing field. Often this knowledge is being applied from other disciplines and there is not 'goodness-of-fit'. For example, when Skinnerian operant conditioning principles are applied to young children or people with learning difficulties they may meet with a degree of success. However, when applied with more sophisticated and intelligent individuals, it is much less easy to predict consequences. Humans are not always as simple in terms of behaviour manipulation as the laboratory rat, and nursing is by definition a complex interpersonal human endeavour. It has been suggested by some that nursing theory or knowledge must originate in the field. That is, a bottom-up approach to theory or knowledge generation is suggested. A good example of this perspective was illustrated recently at an international conference on James

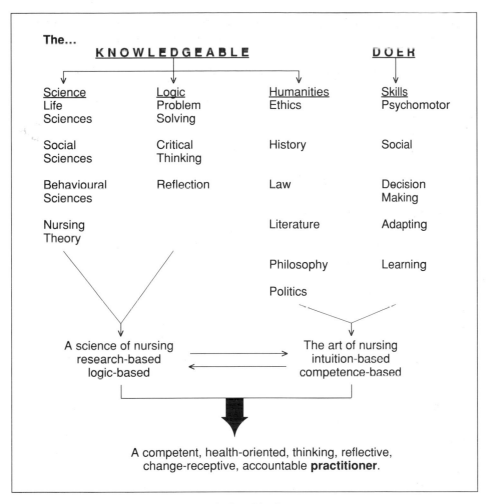

The new practitioner as knowledgeable doer:

The...
KNOWLEDGEABLE **DOER**

Science	Logic	Humanities	Skills
Life	Problem	Ethics	Psychomotor
Sciences	Solving		
Social	Critical	History	Social
Sciences	Thinking		
Behavioural	Reflection	Law	Decision
Sciences			Making
Nursing		Literature	Adapting
Theory			
		Philosophy	Learning
		Politics	

A science of nursing
research-based
logic-based

The art of nursing
intuition-based
competence-based

A competent, health-oriented, thinking, reflective, change-receptive, accountable **practitioner**.

Figure 2 The new practitioner as knowledgeable doer

Joyce in the South of France. The conference addressed such issues as whether or not what Joyce wrote were actually novels in the usual sense. A journalist interviewed Morris Beja, President of the International James Joyce Foundation to find out *why* he was chairing one of the discussions addressing these issues; did Beja who was an expert on Joyce not know if his works were novels? Beja responded: 'No, I'm running the session in order to find out'. This is in essence the 'grounded theory' approach originally advocated by Glaser and Strauss (1967). The idea here, in our context, is that by studying nursing in the field setting and attempting to make sense of complex nursing situations as they unfold, insight and understanding can grow up – a theory from the nursing ground, so to speak, rather than being imposed from without. The relationship of theory to practice is a feed-back loop rather than a linear relationship. That is, theory does inform practice, but practice also informs knowledge or theory.

Secondly, there is a risk that nurses will feel restricted to practising only what has been found to be justified by extensive scientific research. Quite apart from representing a naive faith in the power of research, this is a rather impossible bind. Much of nursing activity has yet to be researched, and this will always be the case as professional practice develops. Some would even go so far as to suggest that some of the more complex humanistic aspects of nursing cannot be researched at all, in any meaningful sense, and must instead be guided by sound intuitive professional judgement. In essence, it is suggested, what we need is a good common-sense approach and the capacity to critically appraise knowledge which may inform practice. The modern health service with its commitment to quality assurance and professional accountability with its commitment to safe and competent practice demands this. Where possible, we *must* of course apply research-engendered knowledge. But as accountable professionals we must be sure that this is *justified*. This even has legal implications, as suggested by Young (1991) when she quotes legal precedent as follows:

'Continuing the thread of accepted practice, the law expects this to be current practice. Therefore, keeping up to date is legally as well as professionally important. In Hunter v. Hanley 1955, the failure to read one recent article or to use newly invented equipment not yet readily available, was not negligence, but if new information is widely disseminated, then it is expected that the ordinary practitioner will read and act on this. Examples are the content of Department of Heath or District Health Authority circulars and might also apply to information widely discussed in nursing journals. For example, recent information on HIV infections would influence the care nurses give and due to the wide availability of the information, this could fall into the realm of accepted current practice.' (pp. 50–51)

It is important to stress here that in the argument for a broad knowledge base the contribution of science and research is not being decried. The contribution of the sciences is significant and vital. Our attitudes require encouragement in a more positive direction, rather than negative 'nudges', as suggested by Tables 1 and 2, taken from Murray et al. (1990). It will be noted from this survey report that there may be rather ambivalent attitudes toward research in nursing. For example, as will be noted from Table 1, while 69 percent of service staff and 92 percent of education staff disagreed with the statement that 'Research is not relevant to the real day to day work in nursing', 64 percent of service staff and over 80 percent of education staff agreed that 'In practice very few nurses use research findings'. This is perhaps not surprising when it is noted, as in Table 2, that almost 80 percent of service staff and over 43 percent of education staff had in fact received no training in research at all. It is of course imperative that this deficit in nurse education is redressed.

In Northern Ireland, the National Board for Nursing, Midwifery and Health Visiting has moved in this direction by introducing a policy statement aimed at firstly training the trainers, i.e., nurse teachers who will be responsible for pre- and post-registration or continuing education programmes (NBNI, 1990). It is also expected that all programmes will address nursing research and the new Project 2000 programmes have been formulated to include a significant research orientation.

Table 1 Attitude to research

	Service staff %			Education staff %		
	*SA/A	U	SD/D	SA/A	U	SD/D
Research is not relevant to the real day to day work in nursing	17.6	13.2	69.0	6.8	1.1	92.0
Research expertise is taken into account in promotion to senior posts	50.6	31.4	17.9	28.4	27.3	44.4
Nursing should become a research based profession	50.4	28.9	20.7	90.9	8.0	1.1
Nurses are too busy delivering care to spend time reading research	43.7	13.7	42.5	27.6	9.2	63.2
Research often leads to real practical advances in nursing care	74.8	19.0	6.2	75.9	14.9	9.2
Research expertise is of value to the nurse in clinical practice	80.4	13.3	6.3	86.4	10.2	3.4
In practice very few nurses use research findings	64.2	14.5	21.1	80.7	4.5	14.7
Research experience should not be taken into account in promotion to senior posts	34.2	27.6	38.2	14.8	15.9	69.3
Research is only relevant to nurse education, not to nursing practice	12.3	7.3	80.4	1.1	1.1	97.7
Most nurses are aware of relevant research findings	31.0	12.9	56.1	12.8	12.8	74.5
Nurses are too busy to incorporate research findings into day-to-day nursing practice	32.4	17.6	50.0	26.1	12.5	61.3
Nmin		500			86	

*SA/A Strongly Agree or Agree   U Undecided   SD/D Strongly Disagree or Disagree

Source: Murray, P. et al. 1990

Table 2 Details of research training

	Service staff %	Education staff %
No research training	79.3	43.2
Study Day	8.7	26.1
RCN Research Course	1.4	3.4
Undergraduate Certificate in Research Methods	0.2	2.3
Postgraduate Certificate in Research Methods	0.6	1.1
Other training	12.0	35.2
N	517	88

Source: Murray, P. et al. 1990

However, we must also be realistic in our expectations. In rapidly changing situations there may not always be an accepted theoretical position, based on sound and accepted research, to guide our practice. Indeed Lindsay (1990) argues for the *need* for a theory-practice gap in the positive sense. He suggests that as theory is directed at extending knowledge, it will always be in advance of practice and there will thus by necessity be a gap. The situation is fluid. Our constant endeavour must be to reduce the gap between theory, i.e., sound knowledge which will inform and enhance practice, and the practice itself. But we can never *close* the gap. In our developing profession today's knowledge base and practice should always be better than yesterday's, but tomorrow's should always be better than today's!

Integrating knowledge with nursing

The argument thus far directs us toward a broad-based perspective in our quest for knowledge. However there is a question of selection here. We must consider which knowledge is legitimately to be included in the new Project 2000 curriculum and, perhaps even more problematic, which is to be excluded. It is suggested that there are three principles which are of importance here: relevance, utility and eclecticism.

Relevance The principle which has to be considered here is that *only* that knowledge which contributes to the study of nursing should be included and that *all* such knowledge should be included. Such relevant knowledge can of course be drawn from the sciences and it has already been recognised above that the life, behavioural and social sciences are essential to the study of nursing.

But it is essential that other disciplines are also given due consideration. Philosophical perspectives which address ethical, moral and political issues and the nature of human caring – addressed by Hunt, and Kirby and Slevin, elsewhere in this volume – have a vital part to play. This is no less true of the humanities. The insights into social injustice and poverty in Charles Dickens' *Hard Times*, the psychological insights into human nature in Joseph Conrad's *The Heart of Darkness*, and the insights into social deviance and psychopolitics in Anthony Burgess' *A Clock-work Orange* would justify the inclusion of such texts in any Project 2000 curriculum. The assumption that only some knowledge is relevant, and that this is almost exclusively of a positivistic scientific nature, is unwise in a discipline such as nursing which depends so much on a deep understanding of human nature.

Utility The principle here, which is closely aligned with that of relevance, is that the knowledge must be useful in that it informs the practice of nursing. This principle presents a dilemma in nursing, where the terms 'theory' and 'practice' are often used. Frequently the dichotomy intended here is between knowledge or thinking – in a fairly broad and non-specific sense – and doing.

In science, however, theory has a rather precise meaning. In this sense theory is the description or explanation of phenomena and the relationships between such phenomena (Stevens, 1979). In essence, concepts (symbolic descriptions of phenomena) are linked by propositions which state relationships between them (Kim, 1983). Such descriptions may go beyond the purely descriptive or explanatory levels, to the level of prediction. Those scientists who adhere to a purely positivistic stance refute the use of the term theory as being synonymous with 'mere' knowledge and reject the premiss that theory should have any practical application.

This has led to a differentiation between pure theory, which is not concerned with practical application, and what Dickoff and James (1968) describe as 'situation-producing theory', or theory which:

> '...goes beyond description and prediction and which must provide conceptualisation specifically intended to guide the shaping of reality to that profession's professional purpose.' (p. 199)

On this basis a number of theoretical perspectives have been adapted to nursing in the form of nursing models which do, indeed, serve a useful purpose in guiding practice. The problem here is that such scientific models have tended to dominate some curricula. This has been particularly problematic where the models have adopted a narrow biological needs, daily living skills or behavioural-psychological theoretical perspective. Such narrow perspectives cannot hope to address the total and complex nature of human caring. Where one or other of these models is adopted as the main or only vehicle for nursing care a curriculum is not only scientifically biased, but narrow in its scientific perspective and often exclusive of non-scientific ways of knowing nursing.

Eclecticism The latter argument leads on to the final principle suggested, that of eclecticism. In the sense intended here eclecticism infers the bringing together in a systematic way knowledge from diverse sources to inform the study of nursing. This implies an integration and synthesis of knowledge. Thus, for example, scientific knowledge can be enhanced by humanistic knowledge which deepens understanding and philosophical knowledge which provides ethical and moral perspectives.

An essential aspect of this principle is that the diverse elements of knowledge which are brought to the curriculum as a whole and at specific points within it must be complementary. It is insufficient to bring to the curriculum a syncretic jumble of unrelated knowledge which serves only to confuse the student. In effect, there must not only be an integration of 'theory' and 'practice' but theory or knowledge must also be integrated within the curriculum.

The social sciences have a particular part to play in this synthesis of knowledge by acting as a bridge or link between the natural sciences and the humanities. This is especially so of that humanistic tradition within the social sciences which adopts the concept of *Verstehen* – i.e. – interpretative understanding through empathy, intuition and imagination – as employed by sociologists such as Max Weber and philosophers such as Wilhelm Dilthey (see for example Outhwaite, 1975). By standing astride the sciences and humanities, so to speak, these more qualitative yet systematic and methodical disciplines facilitate a more critical consideration of the natural and life sciences on one hand and a more insightful appraisal of the humanities on the other.

The social science contribution

This latter contention may justify particular consideration of the significant contribution made by the social sciences in the new curricula. In nursing we have always attended to the individual. However, this has often been in a fragmented way, as in the case of task-orientated care referred to earlier. It also has tended to be excessively 'physical' in orientation, in keeping with the medical model of care many of us were educated and indeed socialised into. A number of researchers, e.g. Bowker (1982) and Wells (1980) have illustrated the extent to which nurses have in the past neglected the social and psychological needs of patients. This was hardly surprising, given the emphasis in pre-registration training on the life sciences (anatomy, physiology, biochemistry etc.), the variable albeit increasing attention to psychology and the almost total exclusion of the humanities and social sciences prior to the 1980s.

The significant contribution of the social sciences has been that of encouraging the viewing of the patient/client in a social as well as individual context. That is, seeing the concerns of nursing as being legitimately *people*, who interact within a social milieu or frame. In essence, avoiding a view of the patient as an isolated unit with a diseased kidney – perhaps even seeing nothing but the kidney itself! However it is rather simplistic to restrict our justification of a social science dimension in nursing to this rather bald statement. The following are some of the more significant ways in which the social sciences contribute.

1   Extending the person-people continuum

That is, as suggested above, promoting the capacity to see the individual in his social context. As indicated in Figure 3, social science is a cluster of disciplines rather than a single scientific perspective. What they all share, to a greater or lesser extent is an extension of the study of man beyond the individual. The message here is that the individual is affected by others and in turn affects those others. When we move to a consideration of groups or people i.e. 2–3 or more rather than the individual case, and when this consideration is conducted according to the tenets of scientific enquiry, we have moved into the realms of *social* science.

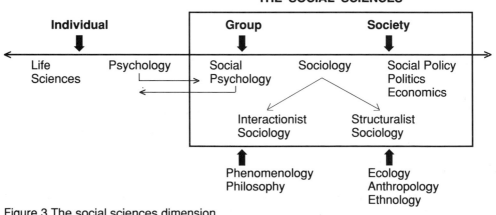

Figure 3 The social sciences dimension

A fundamental problem here is that there is not total agreement among social scientists as to what the tenets of scientific enquiry actually are. In general, social scientists tend to split into two camps. There are those who subscribe to a fairly traditional positivistic science which is quantitative and who adopt in their methodology the survey, the experiment and statistical methods. And there are those who subscribe to a more qualitative and humanistic approach directed primarily at gaining an understanding of the social world as it is experienced by those in it. The methodology here includes the in-depth open-ended interview, participant observation, diaries, personal accounts etc. Statistics and experiments are not involved. As Kenneth Plummer (1983) says, qualitative research is:

'... a peculiar style of investigating and understanding human experiences, a style which simply advocates getting close to concrete individual men and women, accurately picking up the way they express their understanding of the world around them and, perhaps, providing an analysis of such expressions.'

The dichotomy which exists is indicated in Table 3, taken from Cook and Reichardt (1979).

Table 3 Attributes of the qualitative and quantitative paradigms

Qualitative paradigm	Quantitative paradigm
Advocates the use of qualitative methods.	Advocates the use of quantitative methods
Phenomenologism and *Verstehen*	Logical –positivism
Naturalistic and uncontrolled observation.	Obtrusive and controlled measurement
Subjective	Objective
Close to data: the 'insider' perspective	Removed from data: the 'outsider' perspective
Grounded, discovery-oriented, exploratory, expansionist, descriptive and inductive	Ungrounded, verification-oriented, confirmatory, reductionist, inferential and hypothetico-deductive
Process-oriented	Outcome-oriented
Valid: 'real', 'rich' and 'deep' data	Reliable: 'hard' and replicable data
Ungeneralisable: single case studies	Generalisable: multiple case studies
Holistic	Particularistic
Assumes a dynamic reality	Assumes a stable reality

Source: Cook and Reichardt, 1979, p. 10

In more recent times, some social scientists have advocated mixing methods or 'triangulation'. This may involve mixing theoretical perspectives, research design, methodology and/or analysis to avoid the weaknesses of a single approach (Denzin, 1970). However Fielding and Fielding (1986) question the assumption that using multiple methods will cancel out the biases of individual approaches. They argue that the main strength of mixing methods is in choosing at least one method which will address the structural aspects of a research problem and at least one which will 'capture the essential elements of its meaning to those involved'. That is, combining quantitative (i.e. *numbers* and measurement) and qualitative (i.e. *words* and depth) methods in the study of social issues. Irrespective of the particular perspective, the social sciences direct the nurse away from seeing the patient/client in isolation to seeing him/her as part of a wider social world. And, more importantly, they help the nurse to recognise the influence of social forces on health, illness and care.

2 *Facilitating insights into the influence of the group on the individual*

This is mainly a social psychology concern, addressing such issues as attitude formation, socialisation and role theory. One fruitful area of enquiry here has been the idea of the career of the ill individual, how we are socialised into a dependent and co-operative 'sick role'. Another is professional socialisation, how nurses are socialised into being skilled social interactors capable of therapeutic relationships or alternatively cold, distant task performers. Stockwell's (1972) research on the unpopular patient and how nurses react negatively to those patients who do not comply with the sick role or role of a patient, even though this may be a fairly healthy response, is an excellent example of a study of roles, role conflict and attitudes in nurse-patient situations. The common thread in this perspective is how the group or wider society exerts influence on the individual, how the individual conforms to group expectations (e.g., in terms of internalising group attitudes or adopting expected roles), and the consequence of not conforming, e.g. in terms of group sanctions.

3 *Concentrating on the group rather than the individual*

This involves perhaps the greatest distance shift for nurses, who traditionally centred their attention on 'sickness' and the 'bedside'. The idea of looking to the total group – the community or even the society or nation as a whole – is of fundamental importance to such issues as health and prevention. Some nurses, for example health visitors, with a vested interest in health as opposed to disease and treatment would have concerned themselves with such matters. However, for the great majority of hospital-based practitioners the influence of class, poverty, housing, education etc., on health was only given token acknowledgement, if at all. The importance of epidemiological studies and how these can inform and direct health care policy is well documented in medical sociology. What has been given less attention – perhaps even viewed as taboo in some curricula – are issues such as Marxist interpretations of social order and how power is manipulated in society as a whole to the advantage of some and the disadvantage of others. Although perhaps not social sciences in the narrow sense, the reader may be aware of the important writing of Salvage (1985) in the UK and Chinn (1985) in North America which encourages nurses to question power and social order within their professional world.

4   *Concentrating on the individual within a social world*

It is important to be aware of quantitative research which may help us in caring for our patients. Data on housing and bronchial disease, smoking and health, dampness and infection help to direct safe practice. However, insight into the subjective reality of being a dying patient, or a frightened child, or a desolate elderly person entombed in a geriatric ward is also highly important. This is the contribution of the interactionist and phenomenological threads within the social sciences and how these can inform nursing. One such example is Carolyn Oiler Boyd's (1988) phenomenological analysis of the 'lived experience' of nursing a patient in pain – which illustrates the importance of awareness and empathy, and the implications of these for the nurses' 'role-enactment'. Such perspectives are invaluable in preparing nurses for some of their most stressful occupational activities.

5   *Addressing social processes rather than people*

It is often assumed that social outcomes can be viewed as a computation of what the main actors bring to a situation. However, the social situation itself is an important influence on outcomes. A significant contribution of social psychology *and* interactionist sociology has been that of concentrating on social processes and social interaction as much as on the subjects themselves. It is commonly assumed that personality characteristics of individuals determine how they will behave from situation-to-situation. For example, the view that the forceful personality will always force his opinions through whatever the situation. However, in a significant research report, Argyle and Little (1972) found that *situations* influenced behaviour more than the personality traits of major actors in particular social settings. This perspective can help nurses toward viewing social situations as of importance in their own right in a care setting. Examples of 'practicalities' here include Maxwell Jones' (1968) manipulation of the social environment as therapy in the therapeutic community approach and Peplau's (1952) concentration on therapeutic relationship in her model of psychiatric nursing.

In conclusion

This chapter attempts to present a case for a broad-based yet systematic body of knowledge in the new Project 2000 curriculum. Within this context it presents some suggestions on the contribution of the social sciences. These disciplines, particularly in so far as they facilitate humanistic and phenomenological perspectives, clearly indicate possibilities for new ways of knowing nursing. Indeed Oiler Boyd (op. cit.) and her colleagues (see for example Bevis and Watson (1989)) even suggest these as possible ways of radically changing the nursing curriculum, and their 'curriculum revolution' movement in North America has gained strength at a significant rate over the past 3–4 years.

We can perhaps leave these issues with two questions. Firstly, how do we incorporate this complex social sciences perspective into the new curriculum? Our new Project 2000 students, studying to Higher Education diploma level will obviously need to go to primary and seminal sources, to draw on relevant up-to-date research in the social sciences. The small introductory texts, usually unreferenced and seldom referring to research in the field, while so common in the past will be of limited value to these new students who will be required not only to understand but synthesise and apply this knowledge. But how will they wade their way through the mountain of knowledge, such as the social scientific perspectives suggested at Figure 3 above? This question can be answered at least in part by the recognition that selectivity is essential, that only that knowledge which informs the practice of nursing is included in the curriculum. It has been suggested above that, to meet this condition, principles of relevance, utility and eclecticism should be adopted.

Secondly, are we prepared to take the risk in promoting these relatively 'new' (for nursing) social sciences as one of the major knowledge bases of practice? For, make no mistake about it, these disciplines have the capacity to produce very troublesome priests indeed. Remember Essex University and the London School of Economics in the 1960s and the student unrest there. And these were fairly open institutions, not the medical establishment and the conservative health service. We stress in our new curricula the need for a questioning and reflective approach, the need to apply critical thinking to how and why we practice nursing in particular ways. The social sciences have a particular capacity for sensitising students to social worlds and what 'makes them tick'; to in fact question in the most critical way old dispensations. Are we really prepared to take the risk of going down this road? We may perhaps reflect here on the story of the Door of Reconciliation still standing at St. Patrick's Cathedral in Dublin. In the fifteenth century the Earls of Kildare and Ormonde were at war and Ormonde and his followers were besieged behind the door in the Chapter House. Kildare proposed to Ormonde that he open the door and extend the hand of reconciliation. But Ormonde feared for his safety and declined. Kildare took an axe, broke a hole in the door and extended his hand through it – the origin of the phrase 'chancing your arm'.

Are we prepared to chance our arms at the breach created by the authors of Project 2000? Will we make *knowledgeable* doing a reality? Will we grasp this opportunity to push forward the frontiers of nursing in Britain or will we settle for window-dressing and the *status quo?* These are the fundamental questions we must come to grips with as we advance with Project 2000 towards the new century. If we take courage and have faith in our students, the rewards may be great. We may leave as our legacy competent practitioners who – in Oakeshott's words in the opening quote to this chapter – look, listen, think, feel, imagine, believe, understand, choose and wish. This would indeed be a job well done.

References

Argyle, M. and Little, B.R. (1972). Do personality traits apply to social hehaviour?' *J. Theory Soc. Behaviour*, 2, 1–35.

Benner, P. (1984). From novice to expert: excellence and power in *Clinical Nursing Practice*. Menlo Park, California, Addison-Wesley.

Bevis, O.M. and Watson, J. (1989). *Toward a Caring Curriculum: A New Pedagogy for Nursing,* New York, National League for Nursing.

Bowker, L.H. (1982). *Humanising institutions for the aged,* New York, Lexington Books.

Boyd, C. Oiler. (1988). Phenomenology: a foundation for nursing curriculum in *Curriculum Revolution: Mandate for Change,* New York, National League for Nursing.

Chinn, P.L. (1985). Debunking myths in nursing theory and research, *Image: The Journal of Nursing Scholarship*, Vol. XVII, No. 2, 45–49.

Cook, T.B. and Reichardt, C.S. (1979). *Qualitative and Quantitative Methods in Evaluative Research,* Beverly Hills, Sage.

Denzin, N.K. (1970). *The Research Act,* Chicago, Aldine.

DHS. (1989). *A Strategy for Nursing,* London, Dept. of Health.

DHSS. (1991). *A Strategy for Nursing, Midwifery and Health Visiting in Northern Ireland,* Belfast, DHSS.

Dickoff, J. and James, P. (1968). A theory of theories: a position paper, *Nursing Research,* 17, 197–203.

Fielding, M.G. and Fielding, J.L. (1986). *Linking Data,* Beverly Hills, Sage.

Glaser, B.G. and Strauss, A.L. (1967). *The Discovery of Grounded Theory: Strategies for Qualitative Research,* Chicago, Aldine.

Henderson, P. (1990). Foreword in Fisher, E.E., *Behavioural Sciences for Nurses: Towards Project 2000,* London, Duckworth.

Hockey, E. (1987). Issues in the communication of nursing research, in Hockey, E. (Ed), *Recent Advances in Nursing – Current Issues,* 1987, 18, Edinburgh, Churchill Livingstone.

Jones, M. (1968). *Beyond the Therapeutic Community,* New Haven, Yale University Press.

Jowett, S., Walton, I. and Payne, J. (1991). *The NFER Project 2000 Research: An Introduction and Some Interim Issues,* Slough, NFER.

Kim, H.S. (1983). *The Nature of Theoretical Thinking in Nursing,* Norwalk, Appleton Century Croft.

Lindsey, B. (1990). The gap between theory and practice, *Nursing Standard,* 5, 4, 34–35.

Leonard, A. and Jowett, S. (1990). *Charting the Course,* Slough, NFER.

Menzies, I.E.P. (1960). *The Functioning of Social Systems as a Defence Against Anxiety,* London, Tavistock Publications.

Merton, R.K. (1968). *Social Theory and Social Structure,* (2nd Ed), New York, Free Press.

Murray, P., Reid, N.G., Robinson, G. and Sloan J.P. (1990). *Attitudes Towards Nursing Research,*

Occasional Paper, OP/NB/1/90, Belfast, NBNI.

NBNI. (1985). *Syllabus for Part 5 of the Register of Nurses, Midwives and Health Visitors: Mental Handicap Nursing,* Belfast, NBNI.

NBNI. (1990). *Education in Research: Meeting the Needs of Teaching Staff,* Circular No. NBNI/90/5, Belfast, NBNI.

Oakeshott, M. (1989). *The Voice of Liberal Learning,* London, Yale University Press.

Outhwaite, W. (1975). *Understanding Social Life: The Method Called Verstehen,* London, George Allen and Unwin.

Payne, S., Jowett, S. and Walton, I. (1991). *Nurse Teachers in Project 2000,* Slough, NFER.

Peplau, H. (1952). *Interpersonal Relationships in Nursing,* New York, Putnam.

Plummer, K. (1983). *Documents of Life,* London, George Allen and Unwin.

Powell, D. (1982). *Learning to Relate,* London, Royal College of Nursing.

Salvage, J. (1985). *The Politics of Nursing,* London, Heinemann.

Schon, D. (1987). *Educating the Reflective Practitioner,* San Francisco, Jossey Bass.

Stevens, B.J. (1979). *Nursing Theory: Analysis, Application, Evaluation,* Boston, Little, Brown.

Stockwell, F. (1972). *The Unpopular Patient,* London, Royal College of Nursing.

UKCC. (1984). *Code of Professional Conduct for the Nurse, Midwife and Health Visitor,* (2nd Ed), London, UKCC.

UKCC. (1986). *Project 2000: A New Preparation for Practice,* London, UKCC.

Wells, T.J. (1980). *Problems in Geriatric Nursing Care,* Edinburgh, Churchill Livingstone.

Young, A.P. (1991). *Law and Professional Conduct in Nursing,* London, Scutari Press.

3

Integration within Project 2000
(with particular reference to the teaching of sociology)

Gaye Heathcote

Introduction

In designing a curriculum programme to respond to the intentions of Project 2000, a central activity is, undoubtedly, the selection and organisation of subject matter. In choosing, and by implication, rejecting certain elements and items of subject matter, curriculum developers are guided by two sets of factors:
(i)   the intended outcomes of Project 2000
(ii) the concepts and processes that characterise the subject areas or fields of inquiry offered at Common Foundation level.

The emphasis placed by Project 2000 on nurses' understanding of the impact of social structures and processes on the delivery of health care provides a justification for the inclusion of sociology, both in terms of the distinctiveness of its contribution and in terms of its complementarity with other study areas within the Common Foundation Programme. Concepts such as the family, community, social divisions and bureaucracy as they feature in nursing contexts are therefore seen as essential aspects of study, not only because they demonstrate the nature of sociological thought but also because they illuminate central features of nursing experience. Similarly, involvement of students in sociological processes such as observation, information-gathering and the generation of guiding theory based on empirical knowledge, are indispensable elements of nursing practice. The selection of curriculum content is therefore based on criteria of relevance which are themselves informed by a concern to apply skills of 'knowing' and 'doing' sociology to the day-to-day experience of 'being' a nurse.

The selection of curriculum content is however, the first stage in a two stage operation. Once selected, the curriculum developer is faced with the problem of how this content is to be organised, sequenced and presented to students. It is in this context that the question of 'integration' arises, i.e. how to combine the various items of knowledge in a way which is meaningful to student experience and which will enable nurses in training to develop that complex range of skills, qualities and competencies implied in the term 'the knowledgeable doer'. It is this second task, viz. the organisation of curriculum content, which concerns us here and, in particular, the key features, advantages and potential of a Project 2000 curriculum that is organised in a genuinely 'integrated' way. Sociology as a teaching and learning experience is used to illustrate the principles and implications of 'integration' although it should be stressed that the messages are generalisable and equally applicable to other areas of Project 2000 programme.

Interpretations of 'integration'

The terms 'integrated' and 'integration' have been used with a variety of different meanings. In the history of curriculum development, these have often reflected assumptions about the function of knowledge and its ability to portray human experience.

'Integrated studies' has enjoyed a variable status sometimes associated with connotations of 'completeness', 'unity', and positive 'holism' and sometimes compared unfavourably with the 'purity' of 'conventional subjects'. Traditionally, knowledge as transmitted through institutionalised education (such as 'school knowledge') has been compartmentalised into separate knowledge categories which are recognisable as, for example, history, geography, mathematics, physics, etc. However, on occasions, subjects are brought together into broader 'fields of knowledge' which attract labels such as humanities, social sciences or performance arts. The contributory subjects to these fields of knowledge are seen to have shared characteristics which concern particular modes of conceptualisation. One such system, that of Phenix, comprises six 'realms of meaning': ethics, aesthetics, synnoetics, synoptics, symbolics and empirics. Here, symbolics, for instance, is conceived as a field dealing with symbolic structures and including areas such as linguistics, mathematics and logics, whilst empirics is concerned with the phenomena of nature and the universe and includes physics, chemistry, geology, biology and other natural sciences.

'Integrated' has also been used in relation to the way learning is organised. Sometimes this has referred to a particular way of time-tabling such as the 'integrated day' in a primary school. For primary school teachers, child-centred approaches are those which enable the pupil constantly to extend his/her range of experience through involvement in activities which cannot be categorised in terms of conventional subjects. These experiences are often 'guided' in the sense that the teacher anticipates certain broad outcomes but are sufficiently flexible as to encourage a personalised response by each child. Later, at secondary school, 'integrated' may assume a different meaning, referring to a situation where two teachers team-teach on the same topic from different perspectival positions. Underlying this practice is the assumption that a fuller coverage or understanding of a topic is achieved through different subject 'slants' held together by some common ground, yet sufficiently distinctive to provide additional insight to the matter in hand.

Perhaps of greater interest, however, are those references to integration which testify a concern about the possible 'atomisation' of knowledge and the resultant confusion on the part of the learner. In this context, references are frequently made to the need to 'bring about integration in the mind of the student'. Thus integration refers to different strategies which may be deployed by the teacher to link different items of knowledge acquired in different locations and from different sources in students' minds through 'association principles'. A further extension of this philosophy is one that seeks to tackle the relationship between theory and practice by devising activities, experiences and problem-solving exercises for students that enable dynamic and mutually-informing relationships to be established between theoretical constructs and practical applications, between cognition and action, and between 'knowing' and 'doing'.

At first sight, this seems a bewildering range of interpretations. On closer analysis, however, it is apparent that issues such as the nature of institutional arrangements for delivering the curriculum or the extent to which the students are free to develop their own approaches to learning are themselves consequences of the manner in which subject matter is used. Moreover, it is clear that in the context of the intentions of Project 2000, some interpretations are obsolete or irrelevant. We return then to the issue which lies at the heart of this debate, viz. the way in which subject matter is organised within Project 2000 and the relationship between this organisation and the purposes it achieves.

It may be argued that there are at least three major ways in which 'integration' may usefully be interpreted in Project 2000 and that each of the conceptualisations plays, or should play, a key role in the delivery of the programme. The first specifically addresses the issue of subject content organisation whilst the second and third are methodological consequences of this process. These may be summarised in the following way:
(i)   integration as 'merger' or 'association' between subjects;
(ii) integration as expressed through the 'knowledgeable doer';
(iii) integration through students' skills progression.

In demonstrating that the principles underpinning Project 2000 point explicitly or implicitly to the implementation of 'integration' in all three of these senses, illustrations from sociology both within the Common Foundation Programme and the Branch Programmes are used.

Integration as 'merger' or 'association'

It is evident from what has been said so far that it is possible, on theoretical grounds, to associate particular subjects with particular knowledge domains. This is achieved by drawing together a group of subjects with shared characteristics. This process involves two aspects:
(i)   identifying the subjects and distinguishing their common properties;
(ii) making decisions about the principle of grouping and the extent to which contributing subjects should lose or retain their individual identities.

In Project 2000, certain subject groupings are now firmly established in the curriculum. Life Sciences is recognised and accepted as an important knowledge domain in the Common Foundation Programme which offers a study of concepts, processes and insights drawn predominantly from biology, physiology, anatomy and chemistry. In contrast, sociology and psychology may be offered as separate subject components in the Common Foundation Programme but as a combined 'offering' identifiable as Social Science in the Branch Programmes. Thus, for some purposes, exposure to a knowledge domain (Life Sciences) is seen as best achieving desired student outcomes; for others, single subject organisation is considered to be preferable.

Although the reasons for this situation are often not articulated, an examination of the arguments for and against integration sheds light on the issue. If asked why Life Sciences are presented as a unitary body of knowledge at Common Foundation level, a life scientist would probably identify the following advantages:

(i) Integrating science subjects in this way allows a more comprehensive view to be developed than is usually possible from studying individual subjects.

(ii) The explosion of knowledge and rapid social change (and particularly their impact on the organisation of health care systems and nurse education) are increasingly reflected throughout vocational education in a more active preparation of the learner for the modern world.

(iii) The development of personal, social, 'coping' and professional skills that nurses require in their day-to-day work with patients are best arrived at through the study of themes, issues and practical application which transcend subject boundaries.

On the other hand, the sociologist or psychologist, if asked why the two subjects are offered as separate areas within Common Foundation, may argue that both of these subjects have established enquiry modes or 'ways of finding out' as well as different concepts and 'ways of looking at the world'. Students need to experience the distinctiveness and academic integrity of each subject in order to use each effectively as a tool of analysis in nursing practice. Once the essential concepts and process of these subjects are understood by students at Common Foundation level, the combined insights of sociology and psychology as Social Sciences within the Branch programmes offer increased opportunity for professional application at a higher degree of specificity.

It is evident from these examples that quite powerful rationales can be mounted both for and against integration. These arguments concern the optimum balance between skills acquisition at subject level and skills application in the professionally relevant context. They also concern the timing and level at which professional application should commence and the nature of student involvement in this decision. Obviously decisions are taken on such issues by curriculum planners who must balance their perception of 'subject value' and their enthusiasm to induct students into 'their' knowledge system with the professional needs of nurses in training who, after all, are expected to emerge from a Project 2000 programme with a very clear sense of the inter-relationships between theory and practice.

Once decisions have been taken about the value, extent and timing of integration, the curriculum developer needs to consider how the different subjects are to be brought together so as to draw out their common properties. Essentially, there are two integrating principles to choose between – one involving 'merger' and one involving 'association'.

1 The 'merger' principle

Integration can be brought about in such a way that the different subjects (or part-subjects) actually lose their original subject identity. This results in the emergence of a new curriculum study area. Nursing Studies as an academic area in the Common Foundation Programme is, for instance, a key knowledge domain which draws on a very wide range of subjects and part-subjects for its conceptual and methodological matter. Health Studies is another example. This process of merger occurs through:

(i)   the integration of subjects within a particular knowledge domain (as in the case of the integration of science subjects into 'Life Sciences' or subjects such as history, English Literature and Modern Languages into 'Humanities'. This is sometimes referred to as intradisciplinary integration (although this term may be confusing in health care contexts where 'discipline' and 'disciplinary' usually refer to peoples' professional orientations);

(ii) the integration of subjects (or part-subjects) drawn from different fields of knowledge into a new curriculum study area. Technology, for instance brings together components from the fields of science, economics and aesthetics. Nursing Studies too commands an even more extensive territory comprising social sciences, law, management studies, ethics and life sciences. This type of integration is usually described as interdisciplinary.

Whether intra- or interdisciplinary, however, the essential feature of integration of this type is that the subjects cease to exist as separate recognisable entities, but instead became submerged and synthesised into a broader study area which assumes its own distinctive identity as in Figure 1.

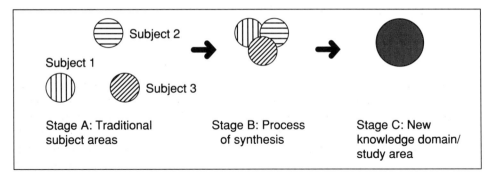

Figure 1 Integration as 'merger'

The key stage in this mode of integration is clearly the process of synthesis. How is this achieved? What are the precise integrating principles here? A study conducted into the nature of integration in 15 school-related curriculum projects of the 1960s and 1970s (Heathcote, Kempa and Roberts, 1983) showed that these 'integrators' tend to be derived from two main sources:-

(i) the 'internal' aspects of subjects, i.e. their concepts, methodologies and processes;

(ii) the nature of the problem or concern under consideration.

In relation to (i), for instance, integration can be achieved in Life Sciences through a conceptual theme such as 'growth and development' or through processes such as classification and measurement. Where ways of 'thinking' and 'doing' common to particular subjects are the operational device, the resulting integration is of the intradisciplinary kind.

In relation to (ii) integration involves the organisation of curriculum content from different subjects on the basis of issues or themes that transcend conventional boundaries between subjects. These themes or concerns may have a practical orientation, as e.g. in Nursing Practice or are non-practical in orientation as e.g. in Nursing Theory. In general integration achieved in this way is of the interdisciplinary type. These principal modes of integration based on *synthesis* are summarised in Figure 2 below.

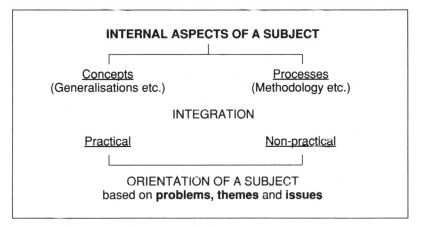

Figure 2 Principal modes of integration involving 'merger'

2   The 'association' principle

An alternative way of achieving linkage between different subjects of the curriculum is by bringing these together in such a way that each constituent subject retains its own identity and logical structure, even when brought into close association with other subjects. Therefore, in contrast to integration through a 'merger' principle, no synthesis takes place. According to one account referred to earlier (Heathcote, Kempa and Roberts, 1983) this does not constitute genuine integration, but rather 'co-ordination' of subjects. However, in view of the widespread use of 'co-ordination' under the label of 'integration', it is possible and probably more helpful in the context of Project 2000 to envisage this association of subjects either as a precursor to integration by merger or as a point on the continuum before synthesis occurs, rather than to dismiss the practice because it lies outside a more narrow definition of 'integration'. We can therefore accept integration through 'association' as the process of linking different subjects (or part-subjects) in a way that effects complementarity and interaction between them but nevertheless retains the characteristics of each consistent subject in a recognizsable way. This is illustrated in Figure 3.

Integration through 'association' can be achieved in two main ways:
(i)   Through establishing a link between subjects on a collaborative and supportive basis. In effect, there is a great deal of evidence in the delivery of Project 2000 in support of this process. All study areas offered at Common Foundation level, for instance, are juxtaposed and sequenced

in such a way as to effect continual interaction and mutual reinforcement, and to achieve maximum applicability to the practice of nursing. This process is also, of course, epitomised by the concept of Combined Studies. Combined Science, for example, is now a widely recognised knowledge domain which links physics, chemistry and biology together but leaves intact the intellectual integrity of each subject.

(ii) Through the choice of a common theme or topic which is considered from the perspective of different subject areas. In the Open University's original Foundation Course in Social Science (D100), the theme of population explosion was approached in a problem-solving way through the separate perspectives of sociology, psychology, geography, economics and politics. This again is a common occurrence in Project 2000. The topic of differential health experience, is explored for instance, through the insight of Health Studies, Sociology and Psychology or the theme of healing through all study areas in the Common Foundation Programme.

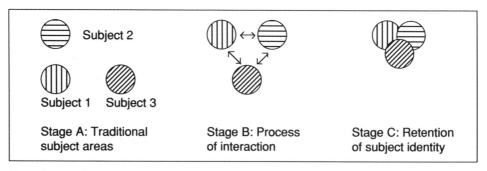

Fig 3: Integration as 'association

Integration as 'merger' and integration as 'association' feature different bases and different principles of integration. The achievement of the synthesis that characterises integration as 'merger' requires, on the part of the curriculum planner, a good understanding of the internal aspects of the different subjects and a clear sense of the advantages of subject identity loss. In the main, the development of larger knowledge domains such as Life Sciences has already been achieved: these are now regarded as almost traditional aspects of a curriculum. However, the content presented under labels such as 'Life Sciences' or 'Social Sciences' is almost always not synthesised but instead stand as illustrations of integration by 'association'. This is because the latter is easier to achieve in an operational sense. It is, after all, advantageous from the point of view of resource allocation for tutors delivering integrated social science modules to take it in turn to teach the class and for each to deal with a particular topic according to his/her specialism, rather than attempt to delivery the curriculum content using one tutor working on already synthesised material. The corollary to this situation, however, is that the students have to work harder to bring about that synthesis in their own minds. This may have perceived advantages as well as disadvantages, depending upon one's perspective.

Integration based on the concept of the 'knowledgeable doer'

The concept of the 'knowledgeable doer' is an overarching idea in the delivery of Project 2000. It is a complex concept which may be unpicked in a variety of ways. In the context of Sociology it could involve nurse students generating their own knowledge about patient differences through the application of research methods 'in the field' and, under observation, applying that knowledge to placement situations. In the context of Nursing Studies this may involve the direct transfer of theoretical ideas into practical situations. Essentially. the 'knowledgeable doer' epitomises the integration which lies at the heart of nursing for it invokes that interpenetration of theory and practice and that dynamic relationship between cognition and action.

So far the discussion has emphasised the possibilities for integrating ideas, concepts, methodologies, processes and inquiry modes. It has been argued that these are 'internal' aspects of subjects which are seen as important for student nurses to acquire or be familiar with. Although located within the parameters of particular knowledge domains called 'Health Studies', 'Sociology', 'Psychology' etc., they are nevertheless relevant to the practice of nursing. Why they are relevant and how they relate to practice, however, is unclear until we come to terms with the full implications of the 'knowledgeable doer'. It is through this concept that we are forced to confront the relationship between 'relevant knowledge' and professional activity and, as curriculum planners, to tax our minds with the central question of how to enable students to 'transfer' subject – based or integrated curriculum content into those qualities, skills and competencies required of the reflective, professional practitioner. The concept of the 'knowledgeable doer' therefore requires us not only to grapple with the problems of knowledge integration but additionally with that of 'knowing' and 'doing'.

Project 2000 offers students a wealth of opportunities for involvement in this most demanding mode of integration. The obvious example here is the link between nursing theory and placement experience although all aspects of the programme are organisationally and conceptually arranged to bring about ample experience in the application of theoretical knowledge to 'real life' situations. The underlying rationale of planned opportunities for 'doing knowledgeably' is that a student can be exposed to actual nursing experiences, problems and issues and, with guidance, be encouraged to apply selected items of knowledge in a way that develops the essentials of professional competence. Moreover, the practice of those skills, once acquired, will inform and possibly modify theoretical ideas. The ethos of Project 2000 is particularly encouraging to the notion that theory and practice are interactive and mutually informing, and that the reflective practitioner is prepared to bring about change along one or both these dimensions where this is deemed necessary for quality maintenance.

Integration through students' skills progression

Finally, integration is often used as a way of describing a student's intellectual progression through a programme of study. This progression is often conceptualised in terms of the growth from exposure to new ideas to a more questioning and analytical response and, from there, to a greater independence of learning involving problem-solving, decision-making, synthesis and evaluation. Integration in this sense is about learning experiences which develop hierarchies of skills and competencies. It contrasts, in particular, integration as 'merger' or 'association' because it emphasises student activity in relation to professional practice, rather than a concern by the curriculum planner to identify unifying aspects across subject boundaries.

Student progression through ever-demanding hierarchies of skills and competencies are well-recognised features of courses leading to professional qualification. In Project 2000 this progression may be achieved through the selection and sequencing of curricular content and by particular teaching/learning strategies and associated modes of assessment. Many opportunities may be provided for individual, directed/private study, for paired learning and the preparation of assignments, for group discussion and group project work. In other words, integration in this sense is achieved through emphasising that students need time for reflection and reflexivity if they are to move towards independence as learners and as practitioners, and time to interact with their peers so that they can benefit from the shared resources of the group.

The most obvious and important example of this type of integration is reflected in the relationship between the Common Foundation Programme and the Branch Programmes. Throughout the Common Foundation Programme, students move through a structured experience of skills development and a progressively more focused exposure to applied professional knowledge. Following this formative period, the qualities and competencies developed during those initial months are further sharpened and enhanced to the point when students emerge as registered practitioners in a particular specialism. Whilst this process clearly relies to a large extent on the curriculum planner's skill in presenting curricular content in an increasingly integrated and professionally-tailored manner, the other major dimension concerns the nature of students' learning experiences and the arrangements made for carefully structured skills progression. This, in turn, involves not only actions undertaken by the curriculum planner but the reflective, personalised inputs from the students themselves.

Teaching Sociology: towards an integrated approach

The rest of this chapter discusses the way in which integration has been attempted in the Sociology Unit of the Common Foundation Programme for which I am Unit Leader. It is described and analysed not because it exemplifies in any way definitive answers to the questions posed in planning a sociology unit for nurse preparation, but because it illustrates the extent to which the different modes of integration examined above i.e.:
–   integration as 'merger' or 'association,
–   integration through the concept of the knowledgeable doer,
–   integration through students' skills progression,
may be used as tools for curriculum analysis and as a guage for monitoring student experience. Curriculum analysis is a powerful strategy for raising a curriculum developer's consciousness of the effect and impact on the learner of curriculum decisions. Similarly, the monitoring of student experience is essential

for the purposes of quality assurance. Through Project 2000, we ask students to make this profoundly complex transition from the status of informed lay person to that of reflective nurse practitioner in a three-year period. We have argued here that this transition may be assisted through the practice of integration. We now demonstrate the attempt to apply these understandings to the delivery of one Common Foundation Programme Sociology Unit.

The first major decision which was made in planning this Unit concerned the nature of the sociological 'offering' to our students. In our planning team discussions, we grappled with the key question: i.e., 'What Sociology shall we teach?' Obviously, students need to be exposed to a selected 'menu' but what should be the criteria for selection and how could this be presented in a coherent, meaningful and relevant way? We examined texts which had been prepared for nursing students prior to Project 2000 and realised that some left a great deal to be desired. It seemed as though their authors had been more intent on mystifying Sociology as an academic discipline, rather than demonstrating that, as the science of society, we can see Sociology at work in every aspect of our personal and social lives. Sociology therefore should be experienced as alive, exciting, useful and above all, of central relevance to the practice of nursing.

The way in which Sociology is conceptualised in relationship to professional training is determined by the extent to which the curriculum planner wishes to retain the 'purity' of the subject area. Essentially, he/she has two options – to create a curriculum which may be called 'Sociology applied to Nursing' or one that may be called a 'Sociology of Nursing'. The distinction can be perceived in this way. 'Sociology applied to Nursing' tends to look like a rather traditional sociology course but with 'bolt-on' examples, illustrations and research findings drawn from the world of nursing. The content is chosen in terms of concepts and processes which best demonstrate the essential nature of sociological thought and inquiry: the exemplification is arguably just a device to 'key' into the interests and orientations of nurses in training. The perceived benefit of such an approach is that the intellectual integrity of the subject is retained whilst at the same time, the relevance of the area for nurses is clearly established. This is, of course, an example of integration by 'association' in which Sociology and Nursing Studies are brought together into an interactive (though not necessarily mutually informing) relationship. The subject identity of Sociology remains intact whilst Nursing Studies offers a kind of 'servicing' function in which professionally related 'asides' support an essentially dominant sociological narrative.

It may be argued that this is not the most advantageous approach to adopt in the delivery of Project 2000. The very nature of Project 2000 and its intended student outcomes justifiably demand a greater degree of integration than that by 'association'. We do our students a disservice if our concern is primarily to induct them into that branch of knowledge we call Sociology and offer them references to nursing as merely a way of holding their attention. What is needed is an approach that is predicated on criteria of professional relevance, an approach which manifestly and intimately links nurse trainees' personal and professional experiences to an understanding of social structures, social factors and social conditions. What is needed therefore is a 'Sociology of Nursing'.

Project 2000 offers a genuine opportunity (perhaps the first genuine

opportunity) for the development of a Sociology of Nursing, a new knowledge domain on a par with the Sociology of Medicine and the Sociology of Health and Illness. The point of departure for such an approach is to envisage nursing as a social process which occurs within structural parameters – societal, organisational and interpersonal. The next step is to ask very pragmatic questions that revolve around the relationship between nurses, nursing and Sociology. Typical questions would be:
- What has sociology to do with nursing?
- What sociological concepts, methodologies and insights are essential for nurses
- What functions does nursing have?' What are the aims of nurses?' In what contexts does nursing take place?
- What are the personal, professional and structural constraints on nurses and nursing?' How and to what extent can Sociology help with these problems?
- How can Sociology illuminate the day-to-day reality of being a nurse?

Answers to the questions provide the curriculum planner with the rationale for the selection of sociological content for a broadly-based formative unit suitable for the Common Foundation Programme. The criteria for selection of Branch Programme content would follow the same process of pragmatic questioning but would relate more closely to the specialised contexts for which post-Foundation students are to be trained. The adoption of such an approach ensures that the curriculum content is perceived both by the curriculum planner and by the student as directly and obviously relevant to professional practice. It also relieves the student of the onerous task of sorting out which aspects of the received Sociology curriculum are applicable to nursing and which aspects of it are present solely as some mysterious whim on the part of the curriculum planner.

A Sociology of Nursing which adheres to these principles is based on a notion of integration described earlier in this chapter as 'integration as merger'. In such a situation, integration arises naturally from the process of pragmatic questioning and effortlessly links sociological concerns with nursing interests. Such an approach does not in any way 'corrupt' or compromise the intellectual integrity of Sociology but rather provides an unchallengeable rationale for its inclusion in nurse preparation programmes. Moreover, it ensures that students see Sociology not so much as a separate subject area but as an integral part of a holistic and, ideally, seamless programme of professional development.

The Sociology Unit in the Common Foundation Programme which we offer attempts to implement the 'integration as merger' principle. We express this to students in the Unit outline in the following way:

'The purpose of this Unit is to provide you with a foundation in areas of Sociology that are relevant to nursing and to help you understand a number of important sociological ideas that we encounter in everyday life. In choosing topics and ideas that feature in this Unit, we have tried to build on the knowledge that you already have about the social world in which you live, and to take into account the images you already hold about nurses, nursing and the health care professions in general.'

The main message of the Unit is that nursing and the delivery of health care is a social activity involving nurses, patients and other health care professionals. To understand the nature, processes and outcomes of that activity, we need to appreciate areas such as people's beliefs about health and illness, differences in their life-styles, their expectations of health care, the hospital as a complex organisation, community care, the status of nursing as a profession, families and other support structures – to name but a few. In addition, we need to understand how sociologists actually find out about these issues and communicate their findings to other people. This enables nurses to develop their own investigative skills so as to enhance nursing practice. This rationale provides a backcloth to the questions identified above and a set of premises upon which to 'frame' the learning outcomes. In the case of the Unit we currently offer, these are:

1   explain the main ways in which sociologists find out about things which interest them;
2   discuss the contribution which a sociologist can make to issues relating to health and illness;
3   describe the features and characteristics of the family and other sources of social support;
4   discuss the ways in which people in society differ from one another, and assess the implications of these differences for the nurse and the process of caring;
5   identify agencies/individuals which socialise people into becoming members of society and understand how this process works;
6   describe the power of organisations (such as hospitals), the effects of bureaucracy and its relevance to nursing;
7   explain how values, norms and beliefs influence the individual's expectations;
8   discuss the significance of the social construction of reality to social interaction;
9   compare the political and social influences on the formation of social policy;
10 understand the cycle of poverty and deprivation and analyse the nurse's role in effecting change;
11 explain how an understanding of sociological concepts may assist the nurse in professional practice.

The above objectives are underpinned by three major concerns, viz:
1   that the nature and processes of Sociology are made to 'work' for nurses and nursing in a way which illuminates professional practice;
2   that there are certain aspects of society and its organisation which directly impinge on the day-to-day reality of nurses and that it is therefore important to understand these processes and be clear about one's own personal and professional responsibilities;
3   that the informed and reflective nurse has a key role to play not only in the system of health care delivery but also as an active participant in the wider society beyond.

The curricular content and learning experiences which enable these learning outcomes to be realised are grouped under eight broad headings:
   The Social Content of Nursing which includes a brief social history of nursing, a session entitled 'What has Sociology got to do with nursing?' and an

introduction to sociological perspectives on health and illness.

Social Structures and Support which examines the family in English and other cultures, alternative family forms, the neighbourhood and community and institutional living.

Socialisation which examines the process and agencies of socialisation in relation to nursing with particular emphasis on education, the professional context, the mass media and the legal system. This area also analyses the concepts of conformity and deviance and societal reaction as labelling, stereotyping and stigmatisation.

Dimensions of Social Difference which studies the origins and implications of differences between people for nursing and assesses the implications of social distinctions along the dimensions of social class, ethnicity, gender, sexuality, disability and age.

Power in Society which offers perspectives on power in general and on professional power in particular. Topics here include medical practice and social control, nursing professionalism and Project 2000, patient power and community action and the hospital (in terms of 'negotiated order' and 'bureaucracy').

Constructing Sociological Knowledge which offers understanding and practice in quantitative methods and positivist methodology on the one hand, and qualitative methods and phenomenological methodology on the other. These methods and traditions are examined in terms of their relevance and applicability to nursing experience and problems.

Social Policy which introduces students to perspectives on welfare and examines the relationship between social policy and the Welfare State. It also studies the role of private medicine, the biomedical model of healing, alternative/complementary models of healing and the part played by consumer groups in policy-making.

The Social Aspects of Nursing Revisited. This final block is a revision block which gives an overview of the sociological contribution to the theory and practice of nursing and an assessment of the contribution Sociology can make to an understanding of health and illness issues.

The pragmatic questioning outlined earlier has given rise to the selection of these eight broad themes. Of course, different questions focused on the professional experience of nurses gives rise to a different set of guiding principles for the selection of curricular content. However, it is likely that the particular content described in this chapter would be broadly acceptable to those curriculum planners who wish to use 'integration as merger' to develop their Sociology Unit within the Common Foundation Programme. At this point therefore we consider the extent to which integration based on the concept of the 'knowledgeable doer' and integration through students' skills progression has been achieved in this particular case-study. In so doing, it is noted that both these modes occur in the delivery rather than the planning phase and that they consequently focus attention on teaching methods, learning experiences and assessment tasks.

Achieving integration through the concept of 'the knowledgeable doer' is probably the most demanding of all the tasks which face teachers implementing Project 2000. The sheer complexity of facilitating a programme of student progression which, over a three year period, enables a transition from the status of lay-person to that of a registered, highly professional practitioner in a specialist area, is indeed daunting. Whilst much can be done at curriculum planning level, as we have seen, to assist students to synthesise subject-based concepts and processes with those principles that can be extrapolated from practical experience, additional measures need to be taken at the level of delivery to create opportunities for the interpretation of theory and practice. Many of these opportunities are created in the fine-tuning and careful sequence of theoretical contributions and practical experience, particularly in the link between Nursing Studies/Nursing Theory and placement experience. The 'knowledgeable doer' is therefore a goal which requires the combined and carefully co-ordinated efforts of the entire Project 2000 delivery team.

At individual subject/unit level, however, certain contributions to the achievement of this overarching concept may be attempted. In the Sociology Unit, the integration of theory and practice may be demonstrated through the role of research and research methods, although obviously there exist other appropriate vehicles in all study areas of Project 2000. In our particular Sociology Unit, we start by considering a range of sociologically researched ideas that ask different questions about the social world and about the role of nurses and nursing in that world. We take student's existing knowledge and interests and focus increasingly on nursing and the delivery of health care as a social activity, set against the structural influences in society of health and illness experience. We then move on to consider how nursing students may generate their own knowledge about these issues by using different research methods for different purposes and situations. Students then become involved in groups in research design at an introductory level and discuss how findings might be used. This leads students from 'knowing' about research and its uses, to 'doing' and experiencing it for themselves.

This process of moving from 'knowing' to 'doing' occurs with increasing demands during the Branch Programmes and ensures an integration of the fourth and final type we have discussed earlier in this chapter, i.e. integration through students' skills progression. In Sociology, as in other study areas of Project 2000, this progression relies on three main strategies: careful selection and sequencing of content; use of teaching/learning methods which enable students to develop increasingly complex skills, competencies and qualities; and use of appropriately 'matched' modes of assessment. In this context, we build in a great deal of provision for student-centred, peer-assisted and experiential learning. Some examples of these methods in practice are: using the library and, as a group, producing an annotated bibliography and essay plan which each individual student uses to write his/her own essay; designing and implementing a simple questionnaire; practising the skills of participant and non-participant observation whilst on placement visits and reporting back to the group; brainstorming; team-building and group work in preparation for a group project.

Conclusions

The metaphors and ethos of Project 2000 are of an innovative initiative which, once translated into a curriculum, is logically and necessarily predicated upon principles of integration. The 'knowledgeable doer' and the 'reflective practitioner' to take but two examples, testify to a mutually-informing, dynamic relationship between theory and practice, between 'knowing' and 'doing', between cognition and action. This relationship lies at the heart of nursing as professional practice.

This chapter has examined a number of ways in which integration may be achieved and has considered strategies at two main levels of the curriculum development process – that of *planning* during which decisions are made about the selection, organisation and *sequencing* of curriculum content, and that of *delivery* during which choices are exercised in relation to teaching approaches, learning experiences and assessment procedures. It has been demonstrated here that both the curriculum planner and the implementing teachers can do much to facilitate students' achievement of 'knowledgeable doer' status by synthesising conceptual and process-orientated content drawn from different subject bases and by re-enforcing this integration through careful decision-making in teaching/ learning and assessment situations. It has also been shown that the integration of theory and practice inherent in the attainment of professional status is too complex and too important a task to be left unaided to 'the mind of the student'. This is not to argue that all aspects of integration should be undertaken by curriculum providers. On the contrary, Project 2000 is equally concerned to create a wealth of opportunities for students to achieve learning outcomes through a diversity of learning routes, styles and experiences. Time and space for reflection, for discussion and for the exploration of ideas are obviously an essential feature of any Project 2000 curriculum.

However, it is morally and professionally unacceptable to ignore responsibility at the level of curriculum provision to extend as much help as possible to students to achieve this desired integration. What is offered here, therefore, is a set of principles for effecting integration at curricular and methodological levels and a recommendation that the resulting integrated syllabus provides a framework within which individual students can, in a personalised way, attain professional practitioner status.

References

Heathcote, G.M., Kempa, R.F. and Roberts, I.F. (1983). Curriculum styles and strategies: a review of styles and strategies of curricluum innovation in secondary and higher education and their relevance and applicability to further education, *Research Report No. 13,* London, Further Education Research and Development Unit, Department of Education and Science.

4

A new curriculum for care

Carol Kirby and Oliver Slevin

The overall goals of nursing education have been inverted. Nursing has developed a rationalist-objectivist model of education as well as an objectivist model of medical science – which means, essentially, that it has come to neglect the philosophical, moral context of health and human caring. Now, at last, we are beginning to realise that nursing education must attend to the whole person and recognise that learning is subjective, contextual, dialogic and value-driven. Jean Watson, 1988.

Introduction

Our motivation for writing this chapter arose from a mounting conviction that in recent years the nursing curriculum lacked a sense of true human caring. While this view is frequently verbalised by some nurses and nurse educators, it has not as yet entered the nursing literature in the United Kingdom in any significant way.

This is not true in the case of North American literature. Since the mid to late 1980s authors such as Jean Watson (1985, 1988, 1989), Carolyn Oiler Boyd (1988) and Sister Mary Simone Roach (1987) had started a significant debate on the need for a care-orientated curriculum. Within what has come to be referred to as the 'curriculum revolution' literature, some of these authors emphasised the need to establish, in a central position in the curriculum, that unique human function they identified as 'care'.

We were convinced that a central issue has to be addressed here. That is, had an imbalance crept into the curriculum, with a greater emphasis on technical procedure and a lesser concern with humanistic caring? Our unease in this regard was heightened by observations being expressed by non-nurses. Sydney Callaghan (1990) a hospital chaplain and founder member of the Samaritans in Ireland, has written of the inability or unwillingness of professionals to share in the pain and anguish of their patients or clients. Perhaps this is understandable. Involvement in high-technology practice may be highly esteem-building, while allowing the nurse to distance herself from a close relationship with a patient. Conversely, talking with, listening to, being with, a pained or distressed patient does not appear to be regarded as important and highly skilled work. In addition, it can carry with it the risk of personal distress and trauma often characteristic of a close relationship with someone in pain or distress. Menzies

(1960) suggested that nurses use social defence mechanisms – such as an orientation to tasks rather than patients as individuals – to avoid these personal contacts with patients and the risk of trauma this might involve. Galloway (1991), a feminist author, writes of her experience as a psychiatric patient. Her poignant account of crying out for personal support, of seeking to have a nurse who would sit with her, just be there, and listen, was disturbing in the extreme. In following her account, it would appear that none of these personal needs were met. While we must maintain objectivity and recognise Galloway's account as anecdotal, we must also be prepared to examine how we as nurses may be failing to meet our patients needs, and why this may be so. Geoff Hunt (1991), reportedly the first philosopher employed as such within the Health Service, stresses the danger of an increasing concern with technology and an emphasis on a market-economy in health care. He suggests that in a general management scenario the overriding concern is cost-efficiency and maintaining minimum standards of safety. And he asks if – in preparing for their role in this 'managerial' health service – nurse are being 'trained out of their moral sense'.

There are of course a number of variables which influence how nursing as an activity is enacted. The political climate and ideologies, the culture of the health care system and the availability of resources are all important factors. But so also is the nursing curriculum and the extent to which it emphasises caring as a central element; or alternatively socialises nurses into a more technical, task-orientated and competency-based approach to nursing work. There is clearly a need for an educational debate in regard to these issues.

Towards a concern with care

> *If caring is central to the health service professions ... the potential and current use of technology needs to be monitored by and balanced within a human wisdom and a vision of humanity which acknowledges certain values.*   Sister M. Simone Roach, 1987

An earlier chapter in this compilation draws attention to the central concept of 'the knowledgeable doer' in Project 2000 (UKCC, 1986). The importance of a sound knowledge base to inform nursing practice was stressed. This is of course a sound premise. However, a problem exists, not only in relation to Project 2000 but in relation to nurse education in general, with regard to the fundamental nature of nursing practice. The questions raised here are:
– What is the essential nature of nursing action?
– What sets nursing care apart from care provided by others?
– Does the 'health' parameter define nursing care, i.e., is nursing confined by a
   health care context?

Kim (1983) defines nursing action as 'behaviour enacted by a person under the aegis of nursing'. While this seems a rather circular definition, it at least draws attention to the labelling of an 'act' as being *necessary* for both subjective and objective endorsement of the action as nursing in a social sense. The purpose of this chapter is to go beyond this by exploring the nature of nursing as caring and consider how this caring can be promoted in the nursing curriculum.

Concern has increased over recent years in relation to the tendency of the first level nurse to be increasingly less involved in the direct delivery of nursing care. A pattern would appear to have developed whereby the demands of ward administration, care planning and the high-technology extension of the first level nurse's role have resulted in those who have received the largest investment in care training being least involved in care delivery. Indeed, professional progression and organisational career structures have tended to lead those who have the greatest nursing expertise away from the direct care situation. It is suggested that the Project 2000 initiative represents an attempt to reverse this trend by preparing a new, single grade of practitioner who is both more knowledgeable and orientated toward applying this knowledge in the delivery of high standards of nursing care.

This chapter addresses the issue of the need for a *return* to a caring curriculum. There is of course a suggestion here that the nursing curricula of the past were more reflective of a caring dimension than is the case at present. However, it could well be argued that as a profession we *never have* addressed in any meaningful way the fundamental nature of *care* and how it should be presented in the curriculum. An attempt is made to examine the essential nature of nursing care and to suggest means by which it can be promoted through the living curriculum.

This must be viewed against current economy-driven values, particularly in North American and European societies. Today, general managers may want safe, technically-competent practitioners and as few of them as possible. Even students are increasingly adopting a value-for-money outlook as a market-place philosophy increasingly takes hold in our society. They want lectures, handouts, hard facts, good examination results. In North America, where the student is actually purchasing his/her education, such demands are reportedly quite forceful. Against such a backcloth, the idea of giving emphasis to philosophical and often rather abstract considerations of 'human-ness' and 'caring" may be rejected as unaffordable luxuries. The position adopted in this chapter is that both these perspectives must be given 'living room' in the curriculum. That is, the curriculum must prepare for:
– (technical) competence, and
– capacity for supportive caring.

It must be emphasised here that while we commence by looking backwards, the purpose is not to criticise individuals or indeed particular approaches to curriculum in any prejudicial manner. Rather, the intention is to illuminate a state of affairs in which nurses became socialised towards a particular perspective, to in fact highlight a situation in which 'care' in the real sense of this word, was not the lived reality. In a sense, this was a situation in which care as a fundamental issue in nursing was no longer its central ethos. There was a shift towards an ethos characterised by technological, materialistic and managerial concerns in practice, which also became reflected in the curriculum. It can perhaps be argued that with the dominant concerns in practice influencing the curriculum and the curriculum in turn influencing practice, such values became self-perpetuating. The problem therefore becomes one, not of replacing one biased ideology with another, but of restoring balance to the curriculum. It is as a vehicle to restore this balance that Project 2000, with its clear commitment to knowledgeable doing and synthesis of wisdom and care, offers a real opportunity for nursing to achieve professional maturity.

The curriculum legacy

Now – to add a note of levity … let's look at it as a drama. The villains are – not surprisingly – men. Their names are Ole Sand and Ralph Tyler. They corrupted a lot of traditional nurse educators and credentialists and are, as Clair Martin calls them, 'guardians of the status quo'.

Virginia Henderson, 1990

Towards technology

There seems to be a general agreement among many that nursing involves both the heart and mind; the term 'art and science of nursing' is one oft-times voiced. The suggestion here seems to be that in nursing there is a need for both humanistic and scientific perspectives as the basis of nursing practice. Wysocki (1980) writes of the unique mix of head, heart and hands that is nursing practice. Our conviction is that the 'heart' element is in deficit and that this is due in some part to the nature of the nursing curriculum.

Prior to the mid 20th century nursing was viewed as an essentially nurturant and by definition feminine occupation. The role of the female in society, going back to the Victorian era and beyond, was essentially centred on the home: childbearing, house-keeping and caring for the young, the old and the sick. The specialisation of some women in caring for the sick could be seen as a natural progression of such gender socialisation influences. By definition women were seen to have the intrinsic nurturant capacity to nurse the sick and the old. And also by definition, this was viewed as neither a suitable nor desirable role for men in society.

Developments were particularly notable in North America, where the rapid advance of medicine and indeed the increasing medicalisation of society, were most pronounced. Of particular interest here were two studies, carried out by Schulman (1958, 1972). In his initial paper Schulman (1958) differentiated between the nursing roles of 'Mother Surrogate' and 'Healer'. In the former role, the nurse's function was viewed as consisting of patient-centred caring and nurturing, while in the latter the role was viewed as being essentially concerned with a disease orientated approach which was procedural and technology-centred rather than person-centred. In a statement which was the subject of much controversy among U.S. nurses at the time, Schulman suggested that the nurse's role would move away from the mother surrogate position and that the basic caring-nurturing function would be carried out by lower-level occupational groups. The profession in America reacted most negatively to this suggestion. However, writing again on this subject some 14 years later, Schulman (1972) argued that his predictions had been strengthened and that the trend away from the mother surrogate role and toward the healer role had continued.

Certainly, looking back now, from the early 1990's, it can been seen that Schulman's predictions were fairly accurate. The concern with extending the nurses's role to take on tasks previously only taken on by doctors was a common feature of the UK nursing literature in the 1970's (see for example McFarlane, 1980; Maguire, 1980). In the UK the more recent issue of the reduction of junior doctors' working hours, and the negotiations on how nurses' role extension may facilitate this, further confirms Schulman's predictions.

Behaviourism in the nursing curriculum

Throughout this century, whether in addressing what Schulman described as the mother surrogate role or more recently in preparing for the more technical healing role, the nursing curriculum has been characterised by a skills-orientated approach. This was certainly true in recent times, when the emphasis in the nursing curriculum has been more towards competency-based training and high-technology.

Pendleton (1991) refers to this approach as instrumentalism, being primarily concerned with procedure and skills acquisition. Nurse educators found a ready model for promoting such instrumental learning in the form of Tylerian behaviourism. Tyler (1949) in his now famous rationale advocated an objectives-orientated approach to curriculum. That is, the curriculum would be centred on a set of educational purposes or objectives. Instruction would be directed towards the specific achievement of these objectives.

The influence of Tyler, and the extension of instrumentalism through the influence of Bloom (1956), Mager (1962), and Taba (1962) in particular, characterised nurse education over the last quarter of a century. In the writings of these authors nurse educators found a new educational technology – a science of nurse education. Curricula became highly structured entities. Course units or modules were characterised by extensive lists of behavioural objectives. The dominant theme was the specification of such objectives, the organisation of teaching-learning to achieve them, and assessment to confirm this achievement.

This had two significant outcomes. Firstly, there was a necessity to be concrete and objective. If something could not be stated in concrete terms and could not in fact be measured, it would be difficult if not impossible to confirm achievement of goals. There was thus a tendency to treat that which could not be measured as non-valid and perhaps uneducational. The result was that the curriculum was filled with the relatively easy (though of course nonetheless important) options – how to give the intramuscular injection, how to pass the urethral catheter.

Other issues – counselling the patient and relatives on abortion or euthanasia, entering the shy adolescent's intimate body space, were avoided like the proverbial plague. The rule seemed to be – 'if you cannot objectivise it, don't teach it!' Schon (1987) is informative in this regard, when he states that:

'In the varied topography of professional practice, there is a high, hard ground overlooking a swamp. On the high ground, manageable problems lend themselves to solution through the application of research-based theory and technique. In the swampy lowland, messy confusing problems defy technical solution. The practitioner must choose. Should he remain on the high ground where he can solve relatively unimportant problems according to prevailing standards of rigor or shall he descend to the swamp of important problems and nonrigorous inquiry?' (p. 3)

Secondly, the pressure to achieve pre-specified objectives acted against any tendency to deviate or explore themes, to change direction and follow what may be more productive channels of learning. There was thus a tendency for the curriculum to be indeed an instructional enterprise rather than a more holistic educational experience. Not only had a set of skills to be learned but a body of content had to be covered in the allotted time. The net result here was that content matter was never discussed or criticised. There was neither time nor willingness to include in the curriculum critical thinking, reflection or exploration of important themes.

The influence of positivistic scientism

In a sense behaviourism in the nursing curriculum feeds off and feeds into a wider 'scientific' influence in nursing. Positivistic scientism has been a major influence in medicine and upon those in the health care field in general. The so-called medical model which dominates health care is characterised by a disease diagnosis-treatment-cure-discharge framework which aspires in its totality to a positivistic cause-effect, experimental science paradigm. Nurses have tended to be in a sense press-ganged into collaborating in this model through their subordinate role to medics. In addition, in its striving for professional status, nursing has aspired toward basing nursing practice on a sound research base. This was interpreted as being a positivistic, objective scientific base. Not only was there a tendency for nurse educators to subscribe to such views, but often their own practice – based as it was on behaviourist approaches – was firmly grounded in positivism.

The outcome of such influences was an emphasis on science and technology at the expense of humanities and philosophy in the nursing curriculum. In effect, the curriculum not only helped to create the *status quo*, but also perpetuated it.

However, a number of nursing authors have rejected the positivistic science model. Chinn (1985) argues that an experimental, cause-effect, numeric scientific method can only be viewed as reductionist and thus of limited relevance in the complex human field of nursing. This in fact reflects a view which also rejects the scientific method. Indeed Chinn (ibid.) advocates that nurses seek a more appropriate method for the study of their discipline – what she terms *future search* rather than *'research'*. It has been suggested by some e.g. Scott-Wright (1973) and Smith (1981), that the way forward may be to adopt a scientific perspective which does not reject humanism. This has involved an increasing interest in the more qualitative social sciences and phenomenological approaches to understanding nursing, such as in the proposal for a human 'science' of nursing by Watson (1985). The American Nurses Association (1980) would appear to go beyond this by emphasising the humanistic basis of nursing as a 'moral art', with ethical principles of justice, autonomy of the person, non-maleficence and beneficence identified as important guiding principles for the practice of nursing.

Notwithstanding the existence of such cautionary voices in the literature, the influence of positivism still appears to hold sway. This is perhaps not surprising, given nursings close aligment with medicine. The modern-day political climate, with the emphasis on a market economy and an increasing preoccupation with cost-efficiency in health care is a second important influence. In this scenario there is an urge to cost everything, including care. This tends to lead to a tendency to emphasise standards which are measurable (i.e. quantitative) and thus capable of being priced. A third influence is the increasing academic orientation in nursing. In the UK, the advent of Project 2000 has seen even closer links between nursing and higher education. In many instances this includes an integration of college-based nurse education into the higher education sector. There is a tendency for nurse educators to strive for academic credibility in these situations. Often this is viewed as being achieved through a greater commitment to a research-based approach to education. This in turn is viewed as being at its most acceptable and most respectable if it is experimental research in the positivistic tradition.

The moral dilemma in curriculum

It is suggested above that a number of influences hold sway in nursing. The suggestion has been made that there is an increasing emphasis on technology at the cost of human caring. The arguments suggest that a behaviourist influence in nurse education and a bias towards positivistic science as the basis of nursing knowledge direct nurses away from a humanistic caring perspective; that nurses are in danger of losing the essential element of caringness which has been taken to be the very essence of nursing – what Watson (1985) refers to as the *geist* or inner self-awareness of nursing as a helping activity.

The blame for this bias cannot be laid in its entirety at the foot of the nursing curriculum or in the hands of nurse educators. However, if these arguments are sound, nurse education is itself at a crossroads. Does it in fact perpetuate the *status quo*? That is, does it allow the curriculum to oppress the profession by socialising its new members into a non-caring, technical, task orientated perspective? In this context, nurse education might profitably draw on the work of Freire (1970) and Post and Weingartner (1971). Herein lie the dangers of nurse education becoming a pedagogy of oppression for those who would wish to reduce health provisions to minimal standards. In addition to these dangers there is also the risk of using nurse teaching to subvert nursing away from a more caring (and perhaps more expensive) path.

At the same time, would it be irresponsible for those who design and deliver the curriculum to ignore technological advances and reject completely a scientific contribution to nursing knowledge? Society has, after all, a right to expect professionals to be up-to-date, safe and competent practitioners. This can be taken to include acceptance of a contribution from research and a capacity to critique scientific findings, appreciate their relevance to practice and apply them as appropriate.

It is argued here that the way forward is (as suggested earlier) to incorporate technical competence and human caring in the curriculum. In the latter regard, this involves identifying the nature of *caring* and addressing how this can be included in the curriculum. Project 2000, and its central concern with nursing as 'doing', offers us a real opportunity to address this fundamental issue. Our increasing awareness of care as an issue, and the coming to the fore of this as a matter of conscience in nursing, now offers us the impetus to move forward with a sense of mission.

The heart of the matter

Energy has been liberated, but into what forms is it to flow? To try the accepted forms, to discard the unfit, to create others which are more fitting is a task which must be accomplished before there is freedom or achievement.

Virginia Woolf, *Books and Portraits*

The examination of conscience, prompted by the necessity to prepare the new Project 2000 curricula, has led many nurse educators – both teachers and clinicians – to say openly to themselves and to each other, something that has been silently nagging away at many of us. That is, that care spoken of emphatically, or practiced in an overt way, is missing, is in many ways absent from our curriculum and its practice dimension. Implicitly nurses care; nurse educators do so too. Care was, and is, intuitively known to be for nursing what yeast is to and for bread. Whilst it may be invisible, in action it is what makes bread rise. It is its life-force. Care is nursing's and nurse education's life-force, is one and at the same time their spirit, their dyanamic, their essential 'will-power'. As such, it must not only be present, it must be illuminatory – awaken us to fuller living, fuller humanity; be the *activity* in which we find ourselves. It is our *quality*, the hallmark of nursing and of its educational process.

Clearly, as stated in our introduction, our caring has not been all that it could or should have been. But we have not completely lost our way: in many ways we have finally found our feet and we do know what we are looking for. And yet, nurse education and nursing has too readily and too often uncritically reflected a society which, 'some people would say is overly materialistic, with the emphasis too much on doing and changing, and not enough on being and accepting' (HRH The Prince of Wales, 1991).

Our past educational processes and the concurrent socialisation into a predominantly hierarchical structure has led, in varying degrees, to boundaries between thought, feeling and action. Thinking with the head – 'using your head' – has been applauded whilst thinking through the 'heart' has been regarded as secondary, if at all. The validation of rationality and the exercise of intellect without concurrent validity of feeling has led to a situation where 'feeling as intelligence' is mistrusted not only by others but also by self; and to a distinct form of disconnection – an intellectual apartheid, contributing to the division of the theory (thought), practice (action) and feeling (sense of being) of nursing.

The separation of thought, feeling and action into distinct entities has been a fundamental source of discord within nurse education in the past. Yet it is the interconnectedness of thought and feeling for action, their integral relationship, that is significant. This connection and the wholeness that is created from, for and to each other, is primary to education. It is such a connection, lived as reality, that is the foundation of a new curriculum of and for care. Thus, caring becomes the foundation of and the scaffolding for nurse education; is the energy that leads us forth, harmonised in thought, feeling and action.

Care is the heart of the matter. How much it matters needs to be said. Nurses and their educators have a mission, a purpose that is realised through care. Nursing and care are one and must be reidentified as such. Nursing care must be voiced in a louder way in our new curricula and be echoed in an essential way in our practice as teachers and as nurses. We must move from a position of neutrality – the neutral body among the caring professions – towards being the activators, the architects, builders and creators of liberated, informed and harmonised lives, and as responders to them. We are no longer 'under the influence' of other professionals nor are we tied to positivistic knowledge and science as an only way. We are firm footed as partners in care and engaged in newer ways of thinking and living with and through constant discovery. Our nursing tradition of caring is not a dead one, rather its spirit is being re-created, a new tradition being born.

A major obstacle (that of subservience to the motives and creeds of others) has been contemplated, in fact lived, and not without a large degree of despair. But we are now taking action. We have to some extent discarded the numbness of spirit, the neutralising force of being 'obeyers'. We have gone beyond the ethic of obedience which had locked us into a paralysed way of being prisoners of outmoded ways of thinking, mindlessly conforming to scripts prescribed for us as to what we could and should be. The primacy of the person of the nurse (and indeed of the patient) had in the past been crushed by the primacy of laws and conventions designed by, favoured by, and in favour of those in power. This situation has inflamed the deep aspiration of nurses and their educators for liberation from bonds which have prevented potentials being realised, personal freedom being exercised. We have firmly rejected the imposed position of being a people having 'half-lives half-lived' and are now saying out loud that 'we must live fully while we are alive'.

However, we are not naive and do realise that we are caring within a particular cultural context – a health care system which has become entrenched in cost-effective, value for money ways. Market-force psychology is permeating the psyche of caring people, is making everything unidimensional. It is asking of us that we provide cost-led care, that we have economic rather than open minds. We must stand firm, be a united force against *exclusively* economic ideals, otherwise we will have overcome a neutralised position only to find ourselves not only trapped and constrained but in every way invalids of governing powers. We must no longer accept having our humanness devalued but insist upon seeing more, feeling more, being more – and caring more. The caring that we insist upon has been articulated by HRH the Prince of Wales (1991) when in speaking to psychiatrists he said:

> 'Caring for people who are ill, restoring them to health when it is possible, and comforting them always, even when it is not, are spiritual tasks. Training people for your profession and maintaining professional skills are not simply about understanding and administering the latest drugs but about therapy, in the original Greek sense of healing – physical, mental and spiritual. If you lose that foundation as a profession, I believe there is a danger you will ultimately lose your way.'

The care he speaks of is not an abstraction, but is that which energises our nursing humanity. It is that which when entered into becomes the heart of the matter for nursing and nurse education.

The essence of care

> *Who has seen the wind?*
> *Neither you nor I.*
> *But when the trees bow down their heads.*
> *The wind is passing by.*

Robert Louis Stevenson

Care in nursing

Care like the wind is invisible. What one sees is its action. What one feels is its presence. The essence of the wind is movement. Man harnesses this movement to his benefit. If we are similarly to partake of and in care we must first identify its essence – only then can we reap the full potential of this essential human characteristic and way of being in the world of nursing.

Nursing is by its nature both a unique presence in the world and a most unique way of being with another person. The sustained intimacy of contact with another, whilst they partake in their personal living activities – often activities only ever performed in the most private of situations – is a major element of nursing's uniqueness. It is these moments, the experiencing of them with the other, that is the love, joy, often the sorrow, but always the dignity and beauty of nursing caring. All of us who are nurses remembered moments when we have, for example, changed the wet sheets from the bed of a woman – termed 'psychogeriatric' and 'incontinent'. When we, having washed and dried her, put a few drops of perfume on her body and onto the sheets, positioned her comfortably and, still holding her hand, stayed awhile; long enough to see vitality return to her eyes, her 'felt shame' disappear. We felt really good – a strong sense of unity with her. Without words she told us that she was 'okay now' – her eyes 'smiled'. Our humanity had been increased. Those of us who were psychiatric nurses have had experiences with people whose whole life experience has been filled with cycles of rejection and aggressive action and who had learned to respond with similar action, who threatened people, made them keep their distance. But we moved forward in stillness, stayed silent but present long enough to sense their fear and absorb some of it from them; eased their desperation. We touched the 'real person' and extended an awareness of each other. We were sources of peace for and with each other. We gave and had peace-of-mind.

These were the moments when heart spoke to heart. When the person of the nurse touched and was touched by the other person, was moved by and alivened through the unity created from the presence of the other. Knew without words the plea of the other. In these moments care communicated itself. These are the experiences in a relationship that defy expression in words. They are the music of nursing – its honour – that must be articulated however imperfectly, celebrated even when words fail to explain. Importantly, they are experiences lived with another person, when to maintain their life they have no choice but to be there, that calls our attention to a unique essentialness and indeed the poignancy of nursing care. The clients whose lives have been altered by, for instance, a cerebro-vascular accident, who have temporarily lost their full power to be *who* they want to be, and who cannot be *where* they want to be, require not only our assistance but our caring for and with them. They most certainly need our fullest presence as a person – our heart, hands and mind and the spirit that is lived through them. This is a time when nursing is expressing its fullest humanity to a person in great need of it.

The paradox of nursing is that it can be at one and the same time the spirit of great joy but also of great suffering; both are moments of very great intensity. However, the 'bigness' of nursing, if we are alive to it and prepared for it, is that it gives more than it takes – our great capacity for a fullness of joy, contentment, fun and happiness is matched with our capacity to listen to and share in the pain of others. The happiness experienced in nursing is witness to Kahil Gibran's (1980) words – 'the deeper that sorrow carves into your being the more joy you can contain'. The joy and sorrow of nursing are inseparable, they are its power and potency – its virtue. Nursing's being, its essence, is lived through:

> 'awareness-creating relationships which are purposeful in seeking peace-of-mind and health for others. Caring is the dialogue between the carer and the cared for and it is inspired through the trust, honesty, integrity, credibility and authenticity of the relationship. The dialogue that is nursing speaks of both the mutual understanding and the mutual confirmation of the other person and of her/his uniqueness and individuality. Caring is, as such, the interior life of nursing – its personal centre.'   Kirby, 1990

Nursing is a unified presence. It can be relied upon to always be there. People can feel safe because of it. Other professional carers restricted by the nature of their work have got to come and go but nurses stay 'with'. As such they are the patients' common bond, a bond that is to nursing its 'commonwealth'. Gadow (1980) who speaks of professional involvement as the unification and directing of one's entire self in relation to another's needs has said that:

> '...the nurse among the professionals is uniquely able to actualise such a wholistic view of the professional. Nursing care because of its immediate, sustained and often intimate nature, as well as its scientific and ethical complexity, offers ready awareness for every dimension of the professional to be engaged, including the emotional, rational, aesthetic, intuitive, physical and philosophical.' (p. 91)

However, it is important to acknowledge that nursings' involvement is not always as has just been stated, and that presence as articulated is not always present. The absence of presence that we speak of is intensely stated by Sylvia Plath (1965) when she says to us:

> 'They have propped my head between pillow and the sheet-cuff.
> Like an eye between two white lids that will not shut.
> Stupid pupil, it has to take everything in.
> The nurses pass and pass, they are no trouble,
> They pass the way gulls pass inland in their white caps,
> Doing things with their hands, one just the same as another,
> So it is impossible to tell how many there are.'   *Tulips*

We are in these instances withholding ourselves, 'indirect one among indirect ones' (Buber, 1919). We are like 'ships passing in the night', are automatons as opposed to beings in mindful acceptance of the other. Gulino (1982) has stated:

'Procedures, the pressure of time, mechanical concentration upon skills, all tend to produce a cold and rejecting attitude towards the client that diminishes his humanity and inhibits the ability of the nurse to develop her own unique potentials. The client and the nurse, like two ships passing in the night, can completely miss seeing each other.' (p. 354)

The context in which nursing is practiced combined with the educational system experienced can and has constructed many of us so that we are as 'ready-mix' and 'ready-for-use'. Thurbon (1991) speaks of 'the system that steels you – and steals you. Your training is not to discuss the things of the heart and this leaves you numbed'. It is the case that many of us develop a psychological and emotional block. That we become as Nietzsche's 'objective man' the one who just reflects the opinions of others, who can no longer confirm or deny from their own perspective. Dilman (1987) tells us that:

'To the extent to which we conform mindlessly we are one of many, and not individuals. We reflect what is outside us and it makes us what we are. In contrast, to the extent to which we make it our own, or reject it, we become what we make of ourselves. But it is what we learn from others in our interaction with them in the course of our common life that makes it possible for us to respond in these ways, to endorse or repudiate, to accept or rebel.' (p. 133)

Dilman's words of wisdom, combined with those of Sartre (1987) that we find our individuality in the life we share with other people, has an important message for nurse educators and vast implications for our caring curriculum. We must acknowledge that nursing's primacy is caring. But we must also recognise that consumers of nursing care have described nurses as being 'uncaring, cruel, rough, thoughtless, mean (and) indifferent' (Kelly, 1988).

May (1983) who spoke of *being* as the 'individual's pattern of potentials', speaks of 'to be and not to be' as reflecting to 'some degree a choice made at every instant', and further states that:

'Perhaps the most ubiquitous and ever-present form of the failure to confront non-being in our day is in *conformism*, the tendency of the individual to let himself be absorbed in the sea of collective responses and attitudes, to become swallowed up in *das Mann*, with the corresponding loss of his own awareness, potentialities, and whatever characterises him as a unique and original being. The individual temporarily escapes the anxiety of non-being by this means, but at the price of forfeiting his own powers and sense of existence ... to preserve one's existence by running away from situations which would produce anxiety or situations of potential hostility and aggression leaves one with the vapid, weak, unreal sense of being – what Nietzsche meant in his brilliant description of the 'impotent people' who evade their aggression by repressing it and thereupon experience 'drugged tranquility' and free-floating resentment.' (pp. 107 108)

Clearly, nursing has in the past failed to confront its non-being. This must be acknowledged if we draw on the experiences of Callaghan (1990) and Menzies (1960) referred to in the introduction to this paper. But we are becoming increasingly aware, facing our weaknesses, and we are to a large extent overcoming our impotence. We increasingly realise that 'events, relationships, or transactions which give a person a sense of identity, of worth, of hope and of purpose in existence are 'inspiriting', while those that make a person feel unimportant, worthless, hopeless, low in self esteem, isolated and frustrated, and those that make him feel that existence is absurd and meaningless are 'dispiriting'.' (Jourard, 1971).

It is perhaps understandable that nurses, alienated from their natural existence as nurturers and carers, would escape into existing as inauthentic beings. This refuge, hiding from oneself, existing solely in relation to tasks and to concepts of role that objectified living, resulted in a loss of personal responsibility with limited ethical concern and interest. The enclosed position was 'dispiriting' and bred, at times, profound worthlessness and a double negation – of self for self, of others for us. And yet, whilst we accept and are to some degree extended by and through our non-being, we can never accept any degree of non-care. We can only ever be diminished by it and, worse still, hurt those we profess to care about. It does happen. We must not only reject it, but stand firm against it.

New roads have become visible. New visions have appeared. We have an open future. We are going forward toward fuller liberation of self and others. Having experienced the 'wisdom of the desert' and 'encouraged by the taste of clear water' (Merton, 1960) we move on remembering:

'The desert is the experience of your own solitude and your own weakness and limitations. It is a discovery that hitting at the boundaries of life is painful and limiting, but also shows us how to relate to others, who are also broken and limited people. We can only relate to others when we have learned to live on our own facing the barriers and boundaries of life. Only then can we reach out to others accepting their limitations and weaknesses and the weakness and limitations of any system.'
Dialogue with Rev. Pat Crilly, Hospital Chaplain 1982–1987, Nov. 1991

The Elements of Care

The characteristic elements of nursing care may be identified as including:
(i)   authenticity of being – realising potentials, renewing being;
(ii)   conscience – consciousness of, engagement in moral activity, awareness creation;
(iii) commitment – advocate with the other, 'with' when the other has no choice but to be there;
(iv)   presence – being with, confirmation of the other person, constancy and immediacy of relationship;
(v)   compassion – the interdependence, feeling for and with, and concern of care;

(vi) empathy – involvement with, acceptance of, understanding the 'way' of the other person;

(vii) empowerment – liberation, freedom to realise potential for self-care, mutual understanding and confirmation.

These elements are not, in their realisation, separate entities but rather are synthesised in the human act of caring. Nevertheless, it is helpful here to consider how each contributes to the caring process.

Authenticity of being

The elements are bonded together in such a way that it becomes almost impossible to separate them for further discussion. They are of equal importance and dependent upon each other. However, if asked, (as we often are), what matters most to nursing, what in fact is its bottom line, our answer is that it is centrally concerned with understanding the other, going out to the other, communicating meaning with the other – the presence of the nurse with the patient. It is the authentic 'I' of the nurse, being with the 'Thou' of the patient. The 'I' of the nurse in 'tune with itself and with others not behind a mask, role, code or ritual. It means relating to other people with the whole of oneself', Buber (1958). The nurse *with* the patient, giving and receiving, is the alive impulse of nursing. This 'giving' begins with oneself. 'Certainly in order to be able to go out to the other you must have the starting place, you must have been, you must be with yourself' (Buber, 1972). The nurses who are in touch with their own 'being', who are their own 'source', can be a source also for the patient. The authentic encounter of nursing is founded upon the nurse who is a personal source, and who can then be a therapeutic source from self for other.

> 'Expert caring has nothing to do with possessing privileged information that increases one's control and domination of another. Rather expert caring unleashes the possibilities inherent in the self and the situation. Expert caring liberates and facilitates in a way that the one caring is also enriched in the process.'
> Benner and Wrubel, 1988

Self as source, is the liberator of self to *become* for others. Caring for others is a primary source of enrichment for self. 'In loving others I am loving myself and indeed involved in my own best and biggest and fullest self interest. It is my pleasure to be involved in the relief of pain of others' (Fox, 1990). To be able to 'go out' of oneself and be for others requires that the person must first find their individuality:

> 'If I cannot distinguish myself from the mass of other men, I will never be able to love and respect other men as I ought. If I do not separate myself from them enough to know what is mine and what is theirs, I will never discover what I have to give them and never allow them the opportunity to give what they ought. Only a person can pay debts and fulfil obligations, and if I am less than a person I will never give others what they have a right to expect from me. Nor will they ever discover that they have anything to give.'
> Merton, 1974, pp. 217–218

The primary command for the nurse is to 'know thyself' and be one's own strength.

> 'In order to gather new strength the strong man must from time to time call home his forces into a solitude where he rests in the community of things that have been and those that will come, and is nourished by them, so that they may go forth with new strength to the community of those who now exist.'
>
> Buber, 1958

This is where the essence of being is, and the depth from which one creates meaning. It is for nurses a very important place to be able to go to, because it is within it that our outer and inner lives meet and from where we find our unity and strength for being nurses.

> 'I do something, I make contact outside myself. I cope. Then, I draw back into myself to sense what to do next. My private world, bounded by my skin, is partly an elaborate sensoric system. It can perceive and re-create my version of, my outer world. That is what is going on as I draw back, even for a fraction of a second from doing.'
>
> Houston, 1982

Connecting with self as such, enables us to be fully with another, but never in an over-involved way. We are our own source of care.

Conscience

'Conscience is a reaction of self-for-self ... it is 'self' thinking and judging moral issues and self taking informed decisions' (Kirby, 1991). Fry (1989) in speaking toward a theory of ethics states that, 'in defining care Nodding states that 'to care may mean to be charged with the protection, welfare or maintenance of something or someone'. Rather than an attitude that begins with moral reasoning, caring represents the attitude of being moral or the 'longing for goodness'. Caring is thus not an outcome of ethical behaviour in Nodding's view, but itself constitutes ethics'. The caring conscience of nursing is reflected upon by Roberts (1990), and she says 'Caring or a caring consciousness, should be inherent in how nurses practice nursing – that is in how they do what they do.... I think we can provide caring care by virtue of a caring conscience'. Conscience is primary to being, a source of being. Care is the source of conscience and as such it is primary to nursing and is manifested through its care. Conscience is spoken of by Blackhaw (1961) when in an exposition on the thoughts of Heidegger he states:

> '...conscience is there in the structure of my existence as possibility, in the fact that whatever I am doing I can identify myself with it or not, and that at bottom I can take charge of my whole existence or not. Conscience is witness to this alternative of authenticity or in-authenticity. It accuses me of living inauthentically, not of doing this wrong, or the other, for authenticity consists in the manner of living not in what is done. And when it calls me to live authentically it also invites me to recognise and live in the knowledge of my irremediable culpability which cannot be atoned for nor remedied like a

71

particular guilt.... Authentic personal existence is personal existence which is resolved, which has faced its sovereign possibility and taken its decision to live perpetually in anticipation of it; apart from any moral achievement which this may be, it constitutes personal existence in its totality which can therefore be known, and when personal existence understands itself it also understands the world: that is Heidegger's professed theme.' (pp. 97–98)

Our caring conscience is not something that exists outside of us, in the clouds or in the heights of profound thoughts, rather it is with us in our everyday down-to-earth actions because it is us. It is obvious when we are who we say we are, and live as we say we do – as carers.

Commitment
Commitment is the dynamic of a caring conscience. It is not a mindless conception of duty nor obedience to other powers, other minds.

'A willingness to live fully one's own life, to make that life meaningful through acceptance of, rather than detached from, all that may hold of both joy and sorrow.... It is the acceptance of one's full responsibility for one's actions; it is the willingness to take risks and to face danger.' Clemence, 1966

Commitment as the moral action of caring requires 'the willingness to enter with the patient that predicament which he cannot face alone as an expression of moral responsibility; the quality of the moral commitment is a measure of the nurse's excellence' (Levine, 1977). Thus the nurse is an advocate with the patient. Gadow (1980) proposes an 'existential advocacy' which is central to committed nursing care. She speaks 'not (of) the concept of advocacy implied in the patients' rights movement, in which any health professional is potentially a consumer advocate, but a fundamental, existential advocacy for which the nurse alone, among all the health professionals is uniquely suited, and which is as distinct from consumer advocacy as it is from paternalism'. She further states 'that existential advocacy as the essence of nursing is the nurse's participation with the patient in determining the unique meaning which the experience of health, illness, suffering, or dying is to have for that individual'. Commitment as a specific act of caring has been spoken of by Roach (1987) as 'a complex affective response characterised by a convergence between one's desires and one's obligations, and by a deliberate choice to act in accordance with them.... Commitment is a quality of investment of self in a task, a person, a choice or career, a quality which becomes so internalised as a value that what I am obligated to do is not regarded as a burden. Rather it is a call which draws me to a conscious, willing and positive course of action'. The committed are united in conviction. They do not kill time, they live it in full accord.

Presence
Presence, the nurse present to, in contact with, the other person is the centre of nursing, the essentialness of relationship. Like most things of immense importance, it is both complex and simple. It is through contact with the 'real presence' of the nurse that the patient can achieve what is for all of us a most if not *the* most

important need, that is, the need to be understood and to feel understood. How then can we say that not present does not simply mean being absent? We have all experienced an absence of presence in a relationship when two people were together and interacting. There was certainly a presence but not one that understood or attempted to understand us. This resulted in, to a varying degree, a sense of emptiness and depending on our vulnerability a feeling of hurt. The consequence of this for a professed caring relationship is well known to all nurses. We have also known the great joy of having been a real presence with the patient. A real presence is an immediacy of person, openness, awareness, freedom of expression, spontaneity, aliveness, someone who adds something by just being there – gives of themselves, welcomes *your* presence, is 'real' to you. You feel real in their company, know that there is no proper way but very many ways. That your way is as important as their way. You know that it is okay to be yourself. You feel understood. They have cared more about you in the moment of relating than about themselves. And in so doing have told you, without words, how much you matter. Marcel (1949) in speaking of presence has said:

> 'The person who is at my disposal is the one who is capable of being with me with the whole of himself when I am in need; while the one who is not at my disposal seeks merely to offer me a temporary loan raised on his resource. For the one, I am a presence; for the other, I am an object.'
>
> (pp. 500–505)

Importantly, to be fully present as a nurse, is not just to be there in fullness of feeling, but also with full knowledge and skill. Nursing presence is then as it should be, a connected person connecting with another person and using her head, heart, and hands. Thus the nurse must have both the competence and the confidence that enables effective judgement, enlivens presence, informs care. Presence as care requires constancy. But a constancy of in – out movement, of systole – diastole. We go 'in' to the patient for a period of time and be fully with him, active in presence. We then 'go out' for a while, so that the patient can experience his own solitude – the enjoyment of being with his own *self*, thinking, doing, feeling, giving oneself peace and quiet, remembering, sorting things out – relaxed in presence. But he must know that we are 'always a presence', that we have only gone out for a while, to come back in again. The nurse is as such a constant presence.

Compassion

Compassion inspires nursing care. It is 'a way of living born out of an awareness of one's relationship to all living creatures; engendering a response of participation in the experience of another; a sensitivity to the pain and brokenness of the other; a quality of presence which allows one to share with and make room for the other' (Roach, 1987). Thomas Merton, two hours before his death said:

> 'The whole idea of compassion is based on a keen awareness of the interdependence of all these living things, which are all part of one another and all involved in one another.'

Compassion speaks to the very heart of nursing, to the openness to love, to life – to all of its joys, diversity and its suffering. It invokes the intensity of image of 'wounded healer' spoken of by Nouwen (1972) who also said that 'the minister is called to recognise the suffering of his own time in his own heart and make that recognition the starting point of his service. Whether he tries to enter into a dislocated world, relate to a convulsive generation, or speak to a dying man, his service will not be perceived as authentic unless it comes from a heart wounded by the suffering about which he speaks'. In its essence compassion in nursing involves not only a concern for and deep feeling of the suffering of another but a going out to the other person, a coming to him not only to share in this suffering but to ease the burden through this sharing.

Empathy
Empathy is the way of being, the involvement that is nursing. The intimacy of nursing's care can only be realised in dignity through the empathic presence of a nurse with the patient. Through the involvement and engagement of the nurse the patient is understood and feels understood. Empathy is an understanding gained with the patient from their perspective – an understanding of their way. This can only happen when we listen with understanding and when we care.

'If I want to know what you're thinking right now, all I have to do is care more about what you're thinking than what I'm thinking.... As soon as I care more what you're thinking than what I'm thinking I will give up my thoughts and I will absorb yours, and I will understand you.'   Solomon, 1991

Scheler (1970) who has spoken of 'fellow-feeling' as distinct from 'emotional infection and from merely perceiving the other's emotion' has said:

'It is indeed a case of feeling the other's feeling, not knowing it, nor judging that the other has it; but it is not the same as going through the experience itself.'

We have all felt so close to a patient in a given moment and as they told their story re-felt their story. We had only heard it but almost felt as if we were experiencing their emotion. But we were not. Our hearts did not miss any beats or rip apart. It was 'almost' and 'as if', but we cared. Carl Rogers (1990) puts the case for every nurse when in dialogue with Martin Buber he said:

'I felt that when I am being effective as a therapist I enter the relationship as a subjective person, not as a scrutinizer, not as a scientist. I feel, too, that when I am most effective, then sometimes I am relatively whole in that relationship, or the word that has meaning to me is transparent... There is nothing hidden. Then I think too that in such a relationship I feel a real willingness for this other person to be *what he is*. I call that acceptance. I don't know that that's a very good word for it, but my meaning there is that I'm willing for him to possess the feelings he possesses, to hold the attitudes he holds, to be the person he is. And then another aspect of it which is important to me is that I think in those moments I am able to sense with a good deal of clarity the way his experience seems to him, really viewing it from within him, and yet without losing my own personhood or separateness in that. Then, if in addition to those things on *my* part, my client or the person with whom I am working is able to sense something of those attitudes in me, then it seems to me that there is a real, experiential meeting of persons, in which each of us is changed. I think sometimes the client is changed more than I am, but I think both of us are changed in that kind of an experience.' (p. 49)

Empathy involves going out from oneself, from one's own thoughts and feelings and getting into the other's to more fully understand them. It is an attempt to stand 'inside the skin', and to 'touch' the feelings of the other person. It is intuitive in that it is dependent upon one's capacity to feel an emotion or situation and to convey that understanding to the other person.

Empowerment

Empowerment is care realised. It is the liberation of the persons so that they have freedom to realise their potential with dignity and in a personally responsible way.

'Freedom is not something man has for himself and something he has for others.... It is not a possession ... but a relationship and nothing else. In truth freedom is a relationship between the persons. Being free means 'being free for the other'.... Only in relationship with the other am I free.'

Bonhoffer, 1966

To realise his potential the patient must not only have full knowledge 'about' but also 'know with' the nurse. The nurse is involved with the patient in a partnership – in collaborative care. The care thus becomes mutual understanding, awareness creation and confirmation of the other person. The confirmation we speak of means:

'First of all accepting the whole potentiality of the other.... I can recognise in him, know in him, more or less the person he has been.... I not only accept the other as he is, but I confirm him in myself, and then in him, in relation to this potentiality that is meant by him, and it can now be developed, it can evolve, it can answer the reality of life.'

Buber, dialogue with Carl Rogers, 1990

Through nursing's dialectic process each person gains awareness of self and in so doing of each other. In talking with the patient, in a spontaneous way, things spoken of can be immediately reflected upon together, verified with each other as to what was meant, felt and in so doing further realisation can be reached. The patient is fully engaged in their own care and holding the reins of their becoming.

Liberation of the inner and outer reality of the patient's world as experienced by them necessitates them being involved in self-caring. Self care has been spoken of by Gulino (1982) and she states:

'The concept of self-care implies that the individual explore his possibilities, choose his actions, create his values. The individual is continually in-process: making himself, seeking his own being. The provision of ready made answers or absolutes only impoverishes man, detracts from his authenticity. The recognition that man is always in-process, always becoming, has implications for viewing the client who seems hopelessly fixed, immobilised in this situation. If the client is not categorised as an object but viewed as a being who resists definition, who is fluid and ever-reaching, his potential for achievement of well-being seems likely to be realised.' (pp. 352–357)

Gulino has clearly made the case for patients being involved in self-care an indisputable one. Our moral sense becomes realised in the everyday activity of nursing care when the nurse facilitates the patient in achieving his full potential; this, in its enactment, is the living process of empowerment.

The context of nursing care

Health orientation

In the preceding section we have spoken of the essential elements of care. These were identified as: authenticity of being; conscience; commitment; presence; compassion; empathy; empowerment. However, many professionals in various walks of life may lay claim to these essential elements – the general practitioner, the social worker, the minister of religion, the school teacher, even the family solicitor.

It can be argued with some justification that what sets the nurse apart is the unique way in which these essential aspects of care are present. For example, in the case of the hospitalised sick person, nurses are present and 'being' with patients on a 24 hour day, 7 day week basis. The injunction on the nurse to show commitment and compassion, to empathise in exceptionally trying situations – often with individuals who others would see as repugnant or socially unacceptable – and to be accepting of and giving to such individuals, is also peculiar in its demands.

Nevertheless, it must be accepted that there are parameters to the nurse's caring function. These are in one sense the parameters of health care. That is, the nurse delivers care in contexts where:
– the health of the well is being promoted;
– the care of the sick is being provided;
– the support of the disabled is being facilitated.

The therapeutic relationship

A second contextual condition relates to the nature of the nurse-patient relationship.

The elements of care outlined above may for example exist to greater or lesser extent in many relationships, e.g., between husband and wife or teacher and pupil. In the former, the goal is one of mutual love and support; in the latter to nurture development and promote learning. In this context, the *nursing* relationship must be viewed as being essentially therapeutic. That is, it must be directed toward the health and well-being of the patient; this must be its primary goal.

Drawing on the review of such intimate relationships by Rogers (1951), Altman and Taylor (1973), Morton et al. (1976) and Kelley et al. (1983) it can be suggested that the essential components of this relationship are:

(i)   Mutuality or consensus (between nurse and patient) about the nature of the relationship.

(ii) Multimodality in terms of interpersonal activities (verbal, non-verbal, paralinguistic, etc) and content (cognitive, affective, etc).

(iii) Discriminatory recognition (where the nurse and patient see each other as unique individuals, not stereotypes).

(iv) Self-disclosure (where the patient's openness is encouraged by the nurse's openness).

(v)   Help-giving, in terms of the giving (by the nurse) and the receiving (by the patient) of help to overcome health problems.

Taking these relational elements and the elements of care described above, the position of the nurse can be viewed as within a unique interpersonal situation. This is illustrated in Figure 1. It is the capacity to enter into this caring relationship which we see as fundamental to nursing. And it is toward the achievement of this capacity in the student that the curriculum should be directed.

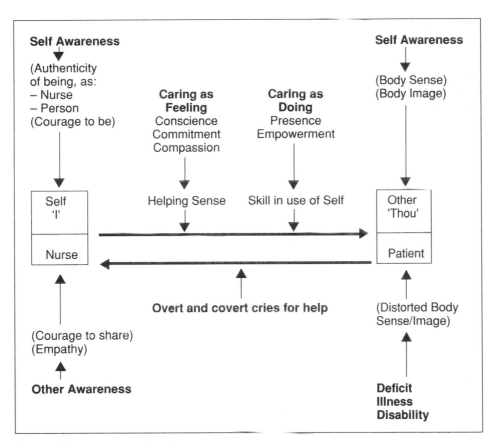

Figure 1 The caring relationship

A new paradigm in curriculum

Empathy becomes technique; the individual, an object; holism, a multi-faceted approach; and humanism, a professional commodity. As human factors are professionalised in this way, a gap between role and person is created. Nurses can and do become estranged from the person that enacts the role. Student nurses tend to lose their natural access to themselves as an outcome of professional role requirements and the conflict between scientifically objective role and humanly involved person.

Carolyn Oiler Boyd, 1988

The rationale for a caring curriculum

In the earlier sections of this chapter it has been suggested that in the past nurse education failed to address adequately the central role of caring in the curriculum. It was suggested that a legacy dominated by a positivistic paradigm, a behaviouristic orientation and a narrow biomedical model of 'care' characterised the curriculum. This has led to a concern with role, behaviour and technique rather than humanity, people and caring.

It is not that this deficit in the study of – and thus views on – man and society has gone completely unnoticed. Sartre (1989) for example, has criticised the concept of role as an instrument of 'bad faith'. He condemns a situation in which the person in a given or prescribed role pretends to be nothing but 'a being for others', acting out a sterile role in which nothing is given of the person himself in the relationship. Downie (1971) extends this idea of the restrictive influence of social role by drawing attention to the schism which may develop between person and role. He argues that the personality cannot (indeed should not) be reduced to the status of 'role' and its limiting sets of rights and duties. The moral sense of responsibility the person brings to a role is an important humanising influence.

The American philosopher William Barrett (1978) has drawn attention to this move away from the personal in a different context. He does this by referring to what he terms 'the illusion of technique'. He argues that in the modern world there is a trend toward reducing all to the level of technology, which seems to be increasingly essential to all aspects of everyday life. In the human sphere he draws attention to the Skinnerian tradition of behaviourism and the premise that people can be prepared through conditioning to cope with all the eventualities they face in life. Barrett, however, raises a fundamental question in regard to how technical man exists in relation to a fundamental sense of being:

'... (the) question concerns the increasing involvement with each other of the ideas of freedom and technique in the modern world. The 'technology of behaviour' after which behavioural scientists yearn, ascribes the most sweeping powers to technique. It is assumed, or proposed to us as an hypothesis, that the techniques exist that can shape human beings completely for all the situations of life. We have only to put them to use and we shall be able to mold mankind in whatever ways we may find desirable – and thus transform the human condition itself. The results from logic suggest matters may be a little more complex than this.... Individual cases occur that are not automatically governed by the rule and that have to be dealt with through improvisation and invention. We are back in the old human quandary again. If we try to flee from our human condition into the computer we only meet ourselves there. The inevitable game of 'choice and consequences' is still to be played out, though on a different level.' (p. 100)

It is the case that in colleges and schools of nursing curricula are chock-a-block full of technique – rules, procedures, scientific models and problem-solving approaches. Yet any expert nurse working in the real life-and-death situation of clinical practice will implicitly know that we cannot depend totally on the rule book and procedure manual; and that, when pain rages or blood is dashing off the ceiling, the niceties of staged problem-solving processes must be waived in an instant and the thing which is known intuitively to be right must be done. Cases differ, the field of practice changes constantly – sometimes in the course of a split second – and the patient on occasion cries out for that which the rule-book cautions or overtly rules against, but which the nurse in that actual situation, in her very essence of being with the patient, knows is necessary.

What, therefore, can all this mean for 'care' in the curriculum? What Sartre (1989) sees in terms of being versus nothingness, Downie (op. cit.) in terms of person versus role and Barrett (op. cit.) in terms of freedom versus technique is fundamental to the question of the essence of nursing care and how this is incorporated in our curricula. We attend, as is suggested in our reference to Schon (op. cit.) earlier in this chapter, to the higher ground of technique and behaviour quite well. But the swampy ground of the nurse-patient relationship – though constantly referred to in nursing texts and nursing curricula – is seldom addressed directly. Care as a word is with us constantly, but no-one ever says what it is, for this takes us into swampy grounds indeed!

This then, in brief, must be our rationale for care in the curriculum. We must recognise that each nurse is a person and not an embodiment of an impersonal role. We must take upon ourselves an attitude that caring in the personal sense is not to be avoided as sentimental and unprofessional, but as being essential – at the very heart of the curriculum. We must not leave the essential nature of nursing, ie, the affinity of one person (the 'helping' nurse) for another (the patient in need of personal help) to informal and unscheduled learning processes. We must instead address it directly, in terms of assisting the student towards ways of coping and being in the caring relationship.

Goals

What then, in a more concrete sense, are we advocating for the curriculum? Here we meet our own ghosts. Having advocated caution against an overly behaviouristic and overly technical curriculum, how can we in all honesty now propose goals in behavioural terms? Bear in mind here that we have not advocated a rejection of science and behaviourism; our rejection relates to the bias in these directions, not their inclusion in the curriculum *per se*, which indeed we see as essential. For, as illustrated in Figure 1 presented earlier, we accept the need for a transactional approach within which the nurse as caring person and competent practitioner comes together in negotiating care with the patient. Nevertheless, we are averse to stating goals in terms of behavioural objectives which may have a tendency to limit growth and self-discovery, and oppress the spontaneity of learning in the curriculum.

The curriculum, at least in so far as it addresses the issue of caring, cannot be reduced to what Freire (1970) has identified as the banking concept of learning – the transfer of knowledge from the active and 'knowing' teacher to the passive and recipient students. It must rather be an approach in which the teacher facilitates the student through dialogue to explore and develop a sense of being as a caring individual, and then to realise this in actual caring relationships. It is a curriculum which does not confine itself to a restricted mode which is in effect the oppression of the student into accepted and exclusively role-orientated and technique-dominated ways of being.

We therefore do not present our goals or intentions in terms of specific behavioural objectives or precise learning outcomes. It is of course recognised here that in the United Kingdom nurse education has a statutory obligation, expressed in training rules (i.e. Statutory Instruments), which impose a legal requirement to achieve specific learning outcomes. But within such requirements, and indeed – we would argue – to assure their achievement, it is necessary to have a curriculum which is educational rather than narrowly 'training/technical' in orientation, to meet the complex yet intimate and personal demands of quality nursing care. We therefore present our goals here in terms of an overall frame and specific themes or unit ideas to be addressed.

Firstly, *the frame.* We have already argued that it is not our intention to shift from one biased position to another. Our overall frame therefore is to ensure that a curriculum will itself frame knowledge and skill within a fundamental relationship which is caring of the individual. This is perhaps best expressed diagrammatically, albeit rather simplistically, in Figure 2.

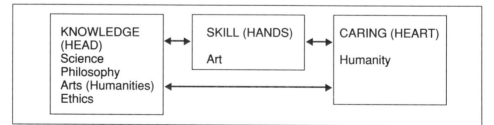

Figure 2 The curriculum frame

Our primary concern in this chapter is with the caring element in the curriculum. However, the development of a capacity to care of necessity requires knowledge and particular interpersonal, cognitive and affective abilities, which may be termed by some as knowledge and skill acquisition. The divisions in Figure 2 can thus only be viewed as a means of identifying the elements in the curriculum; they cannot and should not be interpreted as a rationale for delivering a fragmented curriculum. Whatever the theme, should it be the learning of specific technical skills or the more universal theme of caring, there is a need to integrate cognitive, behavioural and affective elements in the learning process.

Secondly, *the themes* Here we draw on the concept of *unit ideas* suggested by Lovelace (1942). Lovelace suggested an approach to study which:

'divides the materials in a special way, brings the parts of it into new groupings and relations, reviews it from the standpoint of a particular purpose… it cuts into the hard-and-fast individual systems, and for its own purposes, breaks them up into their component elements, into what may be called their unit ideas'.

This could alternatively, though perhaps less descriptively, be termed an eclectic approach, for it involves taking an idea ('unit idea') such as care, or love, or empathy, and using such disciplines as far-reaching as psychology, philosophy, sociology, religion and nursing knowledge itself, to lay bare and explicate the key theme or unit idea involved. Adopting this approach, the main unit ideas pertinent to care we would suggest are:

Self and self awareness	Presence
Person and role	Commitment
Ethics and morality	Empathy
Authenticity of being	Empowerment
Conscience	Relating as being and helping
Compassion	

These unit ideas are in effect those we feel to be essential to the development of a caring relationship as we have presented this in Figure 1. They may not be a complete listing, nor may they be mutually exclusive as conceptual ideas. Our own ideas are at this stage formative.

We would admit here to having our own underlying goal. That is, that our readers will view these ideas and how they are framed critically, to indeed dispute them or point to inconsistencies or omissions. Just as the curriculum must itself be based on dialogue, so too must the development of that curriculum be a live debate among nurse educators.

Towards method

Here again the critical reader may point to a cop-out on our part, as we remain determined to be non-prescriptive. Our intention is to tentatively point the way rather than to identify restrictive practices in the curriculum. In this regard we see the issue of care being addressed in the new curriculum through the study of unit ideas which facilitate ways of knowing and ways of doing. This in essence involves dialogue on practice, experience of practice and a constant moving between these activities. And, of particular importance, it involves encouragement of growth and development of the caring dimension through reflection, as explicated by Teilhard de Chardin (1959):

'Reflection is the power acquired by a consciousness to turn in upon itself, to take possession of itself as an object endowed with its own particular consistence and value: no longer merely to know, but to know oneself, no longer merely to know but to know that one knows … the being who is the object of his own reflection, in consequence of that very doubling back upon himself, becomes in a flash able to raise himself into a new sphere. In reality, another world is born.' (p. 165)

The new curriculum for care requires a process that creates and extends full human vision: the creation of an environment both welcoming and liberating. Its formation is an invitation to the student to discover, discern, justify, be critically conscious of and responsible for her personal perspective whilst appreciative of other people's perspectives. This requires constant recognition of the humanness of each other, of diverse and differing potentials and of the relationship of each person to his environment. The caring curriculum, as in the act of caring itself, goes beyond the transfer or mere acquisition of knowledge and skill toward development of the person. It is a specific approach to personal relating, to personal becoming, to ethical care. Through it care is lived, felt, experienced and understood.

Learning to do nursing – the formation and becoming of the nurse – involves both a journey and a quest. The journey is to one's centre – the anchor that is the integration and unity of one's interior and exterior life. The quest is to enhance caring for self and to perfect the caring that is nursing. Personal and professional formation are one, a connection and interconnection. It is the nurse's person, her insight into life that enables her to become a nurse. The communicative action that is nursing is embedded in the 'life-world' of the nurse. The activity of nursing arises from the 'life-worlds' of both nurse and patient.

Nursing as a response to people's lives is born from concern and respect for all people, thus acknowledgement of the uniqueness of the potential of each person is primary to the provision of a service to those it cares for. It follows that nurse education must be based upon a value system which articulates the uniqueness and inherent potentials of the individual nurse. Its primary aim is that the student will experience the value system upon which her professional practice will be based. Every nurse makes a difference, an individual impact in the world of nursing. The individual nurse matters. Each choice one makes has its consequences for self and others. We are as such capable of making an essential difference to the life of the patient.

The student must be assisted to understand that she does make an important difference and to accept the enormous responsibility which goes with such an understanding. Clearly, one must be personal before one can be interpersonal, be responsible to self before exercising responsibility for others. Only the person who is 'with oneself' can use self as a source of clarification and understanding of and for others.

It will by now become clear that we are not discussing educational methodology *per se* here, as all approaches – lectures, seminars, tutorials, experiential methods, individualised study, etc – may, each in their place, be utilised. What we *are* concerned with is an orientation and an educational process. The mission here is the conversion of the neophyte student into a caring professional. In this we are speaking of a transformation, what some, e.g., Boyd and Myers (1988) refer to as 'transformative education' when they state that:

'Education in an open society has the charge of promoting personal transformation as one of its major aims. In specific terms, education must adopt the end-in-view of helping individuals work towards acknowledging and understanding the dynamics of their inner and outer worlds. For the learner this means expansion of consciousness and the working toward a meaningful integrated life as evidenced in authentic relationships with self and others.'

Method in the curriculum for care must not be so much about instrumental means of instilling knowledge and skills *into* students, but more about how teachers construct *with* students transactional processes which promote care, through an understanding and realisation in practice of the elements of care discussed in the previous section of this chapter. This in essence involves removing issues such as compassion, and feeling, and commitment from the domain of the hidden curriculum or the area of informal, unorganised (and often unrecognised) learning and placing them in a central position as a core to the legitimate recognised curriculum.

As acknowledged earlier, education for care does of course involve knowledge and skills components. It was suggested that in helping students toward an understanding and mastery in these areas an eclectic approach to the study of 'unit ideas' should be adopted. In this context teaching-learning methods appropriate to the study of knowledge from the relevant disciplines and the synthesis of this knowledge in the emergence of unit ideas would be utilised. However, this still leaves the fundamental issue of developing the orientation toward and capacity for care in the student. This is perhaps best viewed in terms of educational processes which run through the curriculum rather than in terms of mechanistic teaching methodology. Some of these processes of particular relevance to the development of a caring orientation and capacity are modelling, reflection, sharing and experience.

Modelling
It is a fact that the nurses other nurses remember from their student days are those who exhibited great humanity and caring or, conversely, those who appeared callous and uncaring in their attitudes. Nurses and nurse teachers are the significant others to their students; they are the people with greatest personal influence. It is therefore important that teachers as nurses are seen to be caring in their approaches to patients and students. A curriculum for care must indeed be itself a caring curriculum – one in which each individual student is valued, one in which it is obvious to each student that care for students, teachers, clinicians and patients is a lived reality. In effect, the curriculum itself must be a model for care.

Reflection
Reflection as a concept can vary somewhat in meaning. This ranges from reflection as thinking critically about practice before, during (as in the case of Schon's (1987) reflection in action) or after such practice, to a more fundamental personal activity. In this latter context, as defined by Teilhard de Chardin (op. cit.) in the quotation presented earlier, reflection involves the capacity for a

83

person to turn in upon himself, to 'know' himself and to develop as a consequence of this knowing. In the curriculum for care these perspectives must be synthesised. The students must be encouraged to think about themselves as caring individuals and to reflect on and attempt to make sense of their nursing experiences in a caring context.

There are various aids to such reflective learning. One excellent example, described by David Walker (1987), is the use of a personal portfolio. As described by Walker, the portfolio was a personal document, no right or wrong ways of keeping it were advocated. It was used to record significant experiences and to help the student 'come into touch and keep in touch with the self-development process that is taking place for them'. It was left to the student to decide whether or not to share the contents of the portfolio with others.

A second aid may be the use of a personal tutor system. In most modern curricula a student supervision system operates and students regularly meet with a personal tutor or director of studies.

However the content of such meetings is usually limited to study advice of a generic nature and/or counselling or pastoral support (see for example Slevin and Lavery, 1991). The notion of moral tutelage, common in old, established universities, is uncommon in nursing colleges. The opportunity to develop a dyadic relationship which might be conducive to a dialogue on the development of the student's caring and moral sense throughout the programme may be of great value.

Sharing

Sharing ideas about caring not only helps the student by validating and deepening these ideas, but also provides the opportunity to learn from others. It is thus not only a reinforcing but developmental process. Such sharing is at its most powerful when it is anchored in issues arising from experience. Where students maintain personal portfolios they may be willing to enhance this process by sharing recordings with their fellow-students and teachers. But perhaps the most significant contribution made by sharing is the extent to which it can place the issues of caring – commitment, compassion, relationship, etc – in the open and firmly on the educational agenda. Through this the student will see that issues which concern him/her also concern other students and teachers, and as such are valid and indeed central educational issues.

Experience

As for other parts of the curriculum, in the issue of care – which is after all the fundamental underpinning of the curriculum – there is a need to integrate theory and practice. In effect, the unit ideas underpinning care must be integrated and in turn be unified with practice. This unity of 'theory' and 'practice', described in Marxist philosophy as 'praxis' is fundamental to the caring curriculum. As suggested above, where modelling is discussed, clinicians and teachers must be seen to adopt caring approaches and must actively promote these in their students. The 'theory' of care, as explicated in its 'unit ideas' must be lived in the clinical situation and also be part of the dialogue in that situation, if care is to be realised.

This is strongly endorsed by Bevis (1988) when she states that:

'Living theory is encountered in praxis, a dance wherein ideas, concepts and theories may arise in the intellect from reading, discussions, lectures, classroom learning activities or in practice. Practice both tests and enhances theory, and theory both tests and enhances practice. Each enlightens the other, provoking insights, altering and changing the form, shape and meaning of each. As the theory evolves, so the practice evolves. In this way, in the truly professional curriculum, each informs the other in the magical whole of praxis.' (p. 48)

Conclusion

Whatever else education may set out to achieve it is its contribution to 'the development of persons' which may be seen as its final justification. What is sometimes referred to as 'individual personal development' becomes the final imperative and beyond that nothing need be said. To challenge it would be unthinkable. Kenneth Lawson, 1979

In this chapter we have attempted to draw attention to the lack of a central concern with caring in traditional nursing curricula. The possible reasons for this were considered, particularly from the point of view of a curriculum legacy which was based on behavioural and positivistic scientific influences. We then proceeded to explicate the essential meaning of 'care' in nursing and how this might be incorporated in a curriculum for care. This involved moving away from preparation for a restrictive, procedural and rule-bound role to a concern with the development of the nurse as a person, a caring self in relation to the patient in need.

It would be a disservice to end our discourse with such a brief summary. Project 2000, the new structure for nurse education in the United Kingdom, provides nursing with an opportunity. We speak of the new Project 2000 practitioner as a 'knowledgeable doer'. This bringing together of knowledge or theory and practice or doing into a new praxis for nursing is laudable.

However we must beware here of the risk of carrying forward old dispensations; of seeing 'knowledge' as positivistic science and 'doing' as instrumental procedure and technique. We must avoid making the mistake once again of failing to place 'care' as the fundamental element at the very core of our curriculum.

The question is, where do we start? The answer must be – with ourselves as educators, for the 'old dispensations' are in fact our own. We have been socialised through our nurse education and teacher training to view the educational endeavour from a particular perspective. We must now move forward with a radical re-appraisal of our curricula, toward an integration of a concern with technical competence and safe practice *and* a concern with humanistic caring.

This will involve for us a process of 'perspective transformation', which Mezirow (1981) describes as:

'...the emancipatory process of becoming critically aware of how and why the structure of psycho-cultural assumptions has come to constrain the way we see ourselves and our relationships, reconstituting this structure to permit a more inclusive and discriminating integration of experience and acting upon these new understandings.'

This transformation of perspectives and transition to new roles and ways of presenting our curricula will not of course occur by magic. Our reappraisal must be a dialogue, not only between ourselves as teachers but with our students and clinician colleagues. Our own hope, as the authors of this chapter, is that for some it will be a starting point for this dialogue and that for others, who are ahead of us in this thinking, it will make a useful contribution.

References

Altman, I. and Taylor, D.A. (1973). *Social Penetration: the Development of Interpersonal Relationships,* New York, Holt, Rinehart and Winston.

American Nurses' Association. (1980). *Nursing: a Social Policy Statement,* Kansas City, American Nurses' Association.

Barrett, W. (1978). *The Illusion of Technique: a Search for Meaning in a Technological Ciivlization,* New York, Anchor Press/Doubleday.

Benner, P. and Wrubel, J. (1988). Caring is the candle that lights the dark, that permits us to find answers where others see none, *American J. of Nursing,* August 1988, 1073–1075.

Bevis, E.O. (1988). New directions for a new age, in *Curriculum Revolution: Mandate for Change,* New York, National League for Nursing.

Blackhaw, H.J. (1961). *Six Existentialist Thinkers,* London, Routledge and Kegan Paul.

Bloom, B. (1956). *Taxonomy of Educational Objectives,* California, Fearon.

Bonhoffer, D. (1966). *Creation and Fall – Temptation,* New York, Macmillan.

Boyd. C. Oiler (1988). Phenomenology: a foundation for nursing curriculum, in *Curriculum Revolution: Mandate for Change,* New York, National League for Nursing.

Boyd, R.D. and Myers, T.G. (1988). Transformative education, *Int. J. of Lifelong Education,* 7, 4, 261.

Buber, M. (1919). What is to be done, in A. Hodes (1982), *Encounter with Martin Buber,* London, Penguin Books.

Buber, M. (1958). *I and Thou,* New York, Scribners and Sons.

Buber, M. (1972). *Between Man and Man,* New York, Macmillan Co.

Buber, M. (1990). *Carl Rogers' Dialogues,* London, Constable.

Callaghan, S. (1990) *Good Grief,* London, Fount Publishers.

Chinn, P.L. (1985). Debunking myths in nursing theory and research, *Image: The Journal of Nursing Scholarship,* Vol. XVIII, No. 2, 45–49.

Clemence, Sister M. (1966). Existentialism: a philosophy of commitment, *American J. of Nursing,* 66, 3, 500–505.

Dilman, I. (1987). *Love and Human Separateness,* Oxford, Blackwell.

Downie, R.S. (1971). *Roles and Values,* London, Methuen and Co. Ltd.

Fox, M. (1990). *A Spirituality Named Compassion,* San Francisco, Harper and Row.

Freire, P. (1970). *Pedagogy of the Oppressed,* New York, Herter and Herter.

Fry, S. (1989). Toward a theory of nursing ethics, *Advances in Nursing Science,* July 1989, 9–22.

Gadow, S. (1980). Existential advocacy: philosophical foundations of nursing, in S. F. Spicker and S. Gadow (Eds.), *Nursing: images and ideals,* New York, Springer Pub. Co.

Galloway, J. (1991). *The Trick is to Keep Breathing,* London, Minerva.

Gibran, K. (1980). *The Prophet,* London, Heinemann.

Gulino, C.K. (1982). Entering the mysterious dimension of the other: an existential approach to nursing care, *Nursing Outlook,* June 1982, 352–357.

Henderson, V. (1990). Curriculum revolution: a review, in *Curriculum Revolution: Redefining the Student-Teacher Relationship,* New York, National League for Nursing.

Houston, G. (1982). *The Red Book of Gestalt,* London, Rochester Foundation.

H.R.H. The Prince of Wales (1991). Lecture to the Royal College of Psychiatrists,

Brighton, *British J. of Psychiatry* (1991), 159, 763–768.

Hunt, G. (1991). *Nursing, Patient Choice and the NHS Reforms,* Belfast, NBNI.

Jourard, S.M. (1971). *The Transparent Self,* New York, Van Nostrand Reinhold.

Kelley, H.H., Berscheid, E, Christensen, A., et al. (1983). *Close Relationships,* New York, W H Freeman and Co.

Kelly, L.S. (1988). The ethic of caring – has it been discarded? *Nursing Outlook,* 1, Jan/ Feb 1988.

Kim, H.S. (1983). *The Nature of Theoretical Thinking in Nursing,* Norwalk, Appleton Century Croft.

Kirby, C. (1990) Caring in a Divided Community, (unpublished essay).

Kirby, C. (1991). A study using the process of dialogue of issues pertaining to conflict within the nurse environment – with particular reference to Northern Ireland, (unpub. M.Ed. thesis), University of Ulster.

Lawson, K.H. (1979). *Philosophical Concepts and Values in Adult Education* (revised edition), Milton Keynes, Open University Press.

Levine, M. (1977). Nursing ethics and the ethical nurse, *American J. of Nursing,* May, 1977, 845–849.

Lovelace, A.O. (1942). *The Great Chain of Being,* Cambridge, Mass., Harvard University Press.

MacGuire, J.F. (1980). *The Expanded Role of the Nurse,* London, King's Fund Centre.

Mager, R. (1962). *Preparing Instructional Objectives,* California, Fearon.

Marcel, G. (1949). *The Philosophy of Existence* (translated by M. Harari), New York, Philosophical Library.

May, R. (1983). *The Discovery of Being – Writings in Existential Psychology,* New York, Norton and Co.

McFarlane, J.K. (1980). *Essays on Nursing,* London, King's Fund Centre.

Menzies, I.E.P. (1960). *The Functioning of Social Systems as a Defence Against Anxiety,* London, Tavistock Publications.

Merton, T. (1960). *The Wisdom of the Desert,* London, Sheldon Press.

Merton, T. (1974). *No Man is an Island,* London, Burns and Oats.

Mezirow, J. (1981). A critical theory of adult learning and education, *Adult Education (Journal of Adult Education Association of the USA),* 32, 1, 3–24.

Morton, T.L., Alexander, J. and Altman, I. (1976). Communication and relationship definition.

in G.R. Miller (Ed.), *Explorations in Interpersonal Communication,* London, Sage Publications.

Nouwen. (1972). *The Wounded Healer, Ministry in Contemporary Society,* New York, Doubleday.

Pendleton, S. (1991). Curriculum planning in nursing education: towards the year 2000, in S. Pendleton and A. Myles (Eds.), *Curriculum Planning in Nursing Education: Practical Applications,* London, Edward Arnold.

Plath, S. (1965). Tulips, in S. Plath, *Ariel – Poems by Sylvia Plath,* London, Faber.

Post, N. and Weingartner, C. (1971). *Teaching as a Subversive Activity,* Harmondsworth, Penguin.

Roach, Sister M. Simone (1987). *The Human Act of Caring,* Ottowa, Canadian Hospital Association.

Roberts, J.E. (1990). Uncovering hidden caring, *Nursing Outlook,* 38, 2, 67–69.

Rogers, C. (1951). *Client-centred Therapy,* Boston, Houghton Mifflin.

Rogers, C. (1990). *Carl Rogers' Dialogues,* London, Constable.

Sartre, J-P. (1987). – quoted in A. Cohen-Solal, *Sartre – A Life,* London, Heinemann.

Sartre, J-P. (1989). *Being and Nothingness,* London, Routledge.

Scheler, M. (1970). *The Nature of Sympathy,* (translated by P. Heath), Hamdon, Archon Books.

Schon, D. (1987). *Educating the Reflective Practitioner,* San Francisco, Jossey Bass.

Schulman, S. (1958). Basic functional roles in nursing: mother surrogate and healer, in E. G. Jaco (Ed.), *Patients, Physicians and Illness: Sourcebook in Behavioral Science and Medicine,* New York, Free Press.

Schulman, S. (1972). Mother-surrogate – after a decade, in E. G. Jaco (Ed.), *Patients,*

Physicians and Illness: a Sourcebook in Behavioral Science and Medicine (2nd edition), London, Collier-Macmillan.

Scott-Wright, M. (1973). Nursing and universities, Inaugural lecture No. 54, University of Edinburgh.

Slevin, O.D'A. and Lavery, M.C. (1991). Self-directed learning and student supervision, *Nurse Education Today,* 11, 368–377.

Smith, J.P. (1981). *Nursing Science in Nursing Practice,* London, Butterworth.

Solomon, P. (1991). Paul Solomon speaks on spiritual roots and the journey to wholeness, *Human Potential Magazine,* 16, 3, 28–32.

Taba, H. (1962). *Curriculum Development – Theory and Practice,* New York, Harcourt, Brace and World.

Teilhard de Chardin, P. (1959). *The Phenomenon of Man,* London, Collins.

Thurbon, C. (1991). In dialogue with Penny Perrick, *Sunday Times,* 8 September 1991.

Tyler, R. (1949). *Basic Principles of Curriculum Instruction,* Chicago, University of Chicago Press.

UKCC. (1986). *Project 2000: a New Preparation for Practice,* London, UKCC.

Walker, D. (1987). Writing and reflection, in D. Boud, R. Keogh and D. Walker (Eds.), *Reflection: Turning Experience into Learning,* London, Kogan Page.

Watson, J. (1985). *Nursing: The Philosophy and Science of Caring,* Boulder, Colorado, Associated University Press.

Watson, J. (1988). A case study: curriculum in transition, in *Curriculum Revolution: Mandate for Change,* New York, National League for Nursing.

Watson, J. (1989). A new paradigm of curriculum development, in E. O. Bevis and J. Watson (Eds.), *Toward a Caring Curriculum: A New Pedagogy for Nursing,* New York, National League for Nursing.

Wysocki, R. (1980). Evaluation of student clinical performance, *Australian Nurses Journal,* 10, 5, 42–43.

5

Project 2000:
Ethics, ambivalence and ideology

Geoffrey Hunt

'We can't afford to think in that way'

Recently I was asked to introduce Ethics to a group of qualified and experienced nurses. I began by asking them to give me some 'scientific' terms. There was hardly any hesitation. 'Gastric', 'pulmonary', 'embolism', 'nephritis', 'pharynx', 'dialysis' were proffered. I nodded, and more and more terms tumbled out. The class was enjoying itself.

I then asked for some 'technical' terms which might be used in describing everyday nursing procedures. They were really into the swing of it now: 'wound management', 'enema', 'catheter', 'hygiene', 'traction', 'ward round', 'mobility', 'bed sore', 'skill mix', 'stoma care', 'syringe'.

Then I asked if they could provide me with some moral or ethical terms relevant to nursing. There was a long silence. 'You do know what I mean by 'moral' and 'ethical'?' I asked, hoping I did not sound patronising. 'Oh, yes', they said. But the problem was relating morality to nursing. I coaxed them: 'Give me any word which describes what a nurse ought or ought not do, or the character of a nurse or patient, or a situation in which a question of right and wrong arises.'

Someone came up with a term: 'Stress'. Another two followed: 'communication', 'counselling'. Do these words really belong to our *moral* vocabulary? I asked. Aeroplane wings and bridge cantilevers are subject to stress; computers and robots communicate; and counselling is generally thought to rest on the science of psychology.

The class was completely stuck. I changed tack. What do you look for in a good friend? I asked. A change of weather came over the faces before me. The sun was appearing. Mentally they were stepping out of their uniforms. 'Honesty', said one. 'Loyalty', said another. 'An ability to keep my secrets, respect for me, understanding, trust, caring about me, being there when I need him/her, sharing problems.' They now had no hesitation whatsoever.

'Don't any of these have anything to do with nursing patients?' I now asked. A collective 'Oh, I see!' rippled across the classroom. One nurse explained: 'We're just not used to thinking in that way.' The cynical rejoinder came from another: 'We can't afford to think in that way!' I then suggested we look at health care from the point of view of the *patients*. All of us in the room had been or would be patients at some time. Then it was as clear as day to everyone that nurses could not afford *not* to think in that way.

Here, then, is the product of a century of nurse education. Here is the end result of a hierarchical and technocratic health care system, one which voids health care of its moral ground.

Progress in health care now largely requires not medical discovery but *ethical rediscovery*. I say rediscovery, because I believe that the principal task of Ethics is to remind us of what has been pushed out of our lives by the over-extension of the science and technology which serve rationalising bureaucracies. All too often, what we know very well in our encounters with our loved ones, and enemies, we put aside as irrelevant as soon as we put on our uniforms. Even the language of morality is often substituted with the misleading and alienating language of psychology and management – as my opening anecdote shows.

Project 2000 may – I do not say it necessarily will – provide an opportunity to put the morally responsible nurse, midwife and health visitor at the forefront of the transformation which health care so urgently needs for the next century.

New right ideology

Crisis and the Establishment

We live very much in the past in the U.K., and find it hard to shake ourselves loose. When old ideas, old systems, old institutions no longer work, so reluctant are we to give them up that we are prone to lapse into cynicism, sarcastic humour and self-centred escapism rather than cooperate, innovate and challenge. We also tend to look to the past for old solutions.

Worse, it is a deeply ingrained attitude in this country that 'authorities' should lead, while the rest of us unquestioningly follow. The Establishment is assumed to know what is in the 'national interest', and can be trusted. Experts are in control. Doctors, blessed with an uncanny scientific insight called 'clinical judgment', know what is in the best interest of the patient, managers know how to employ resources most efficiently, lawyers defend us with a legal system which is supposedly held up as a model by the rest of the world, we are so civilised and decent that we do not need a constitution or a Bill of Rights, and gentlemanly behaviour prevails.

Nursing has suffered, more than most professions, from the stranglehold of complacent authoritarianism and public passivity. Yet nurses have known for a long time that mere competence in a range of tasks and a willing subservience to medical and managerial instructions leave a very great deal to be desired. They have never had the moral and political freedom to act on this knowledge. The recent initiatives of the statutory bodies in reconceiving nurse education and professional responsibility and conduct are making anachronistic and intolerable the continuation of a health care system which, in its very structures and assumptions, still prevents or discourages the moral liberation of nurses.

Since nurses cannot expect much outside initiative in breaking the fetters on their freedom – not from health authorities, or hospital management or Government, nor even apparently from their unions – they may have to take the initiative themselves. Project 2000, I will argue, provides some opportunities for doing just this in so far as it embraces ethics and the law in the new nurse education. I say 'opportunities' because Project 2000 is somewhat ambivalent, and does not fully recognise the economic and political context in which it will be implemented.

Conflict of ideal and reality

There has always been a glaring discrepancy between the ideals of nursing and the realities of nursing practice with all its constraints. If the nursing profession as a whole remains unaware of the character and significance of current developments (and non-developments) in the health care delivery system it will continue to stand by and observe powerlessly as that discrepancy takes yet another new form, indeed a deeper and more pernicious form than ever.

The 1986 *Report of the Project 2000 Group* [1] states that 'The new directions of development in education and training and in professional conduct are interlinked. Together they add up to a new model of professional regulation and they affirm a more mature approach to what a professional is and should do ...' (p. 33). Indeed it is salutary to read the elaboration by the United Kingdom Central Council for Nursing, Midwifery and Health Visiting (UKCC) of its Professional Code in its 1989 document *Exercising Accountability* [2] together with the Project 2000 Report.

However, since neither document fully appreciates the distinction between moral responsibility and professional ethics (which I discuss below), they leave unresolved the question of *implementation* in the contemporary health care delivery environment. A question I will be very concerned with in this chapter is that of closing the gap between the new ideals and the actual practice of nursing in an unchanging hierarchy and the new market-led environment. This is especially important when the ideals themselves are at certain crucial points ambivalently conceived and expressed.

To give an example. The UKCC's ethical code in many ways requires changes in practice which run counter to the interests and power of the medical-managerial hierarchy; but there are few, if any, signs that the hierarchy will change to accommodate such changes. Thus, *Exercising Accountability*, gives nurses a professional responsibility for ensuring that informed consent has been obtained from patients. It states that the nurse 'might decide not to co-operate with a procedure if convinced that the decision to agree to it being performed was not truly informed' (Section D. 3). The code recommends that a nurse recall a doctor to give the information again if a discussion with the patient reveals that the doctor has not been understood.

Yet how many concrete steps have been taken by government, health authorities and hospital managers to institute practical procedures and safeguards for nurses who enact this codified responsibility? Without such steps can we envisage a self-regulating nursing environment in which nurses encourage each other to intervene in cases of invalid consent and take to task those who do not intervene?

A system in crisis poses conflicting necessities: it needs to extend the responsibilities of nurses, but it also needs to do so without threatening the existing power bases.

Project 2000, and its concern with moral and ethical matters, is not an isolated development. Already there has been a burgeoning of new areas of thought such as bio-ethics and medical ethics. The social and institutional factors which have given rise to these new areas are also having their impact on nursing, midwifery and health visiting.

There is a global crisis in health care systems which has thrown the political, economic and administrative *status quo* into turmoil. Neither the state bureaucratic system nor the private delivery system work very well. Medical manufacturing corporations (especially pharmaceutical companies), medical consultants and, increasingly, managers have too much power and influence. The new technological developments which go hand-in-hand with this power, such as 'genetic engineering' and 'reproductive technology', have created new moral and political issues and dilemmas.

Recent movements for social rights, and a greater knowledge of health matters on the part of the general public, have presented challenges to the Health Care Establishment. A pervasive intellectual crisis in medicine, which arises from the profession's ignorance of 20th century changes in the scientific paradigm, has so far produced more defensiveness, more arrogance and more tenacity in clinging to outdated modes of thought about human health and wellbeing.

There is not a great deal of evidence that nurse educators are attempting to understand Project 2000 *in the political and economic context* of our times, yet such an understanding is urgently needed. Indeed, the project has to be seen in the light of contemporary ideological currents, particularly that of the New Right ([3]). It has to be recognised that the ideology of the New Right, which has been in power for 13 years, is working against Project 2000. The ideology looks to the past for its model of society, while the project innovatively looks to the future.

I will now take up three themes in relation to the official ideology of the eighties and early nineties, and show how paradoxical it is that the ideals and recommendations of Project 2000 should have emerged at such an unaccommodating time. The three themes are: patients and consumers; the community; confidentiality and secrecy.

Patients, consumers and the unwell

The current transformation of the patient into the consumer is one of the disturbing signs of a deepening disempowerment of the needy. The patient, who never had any real power anyway, was at least recognised as a citizen who had rights as well as duties or obligations. Among the rights was a right to welfare according to need, and among the obligations was that of paying tax to support the needy.

The New Right ideology puts all the emphasis on obligations and neglects rights. Rights have been narrowed into consumer rights: a fair price, unadulterated goods, contractual agreements.

If this ideology is successful, where would the shift in our conception of the patient put nursing? What is the difference between the nurse in relation to the patient and the nurse in relation to the consumer? In fact we have to ask whether 'nurse' can be defined at all in relation to the consumer. Nursing has always taken part of its meaning from the perception of certain classes of people as 'patients'. I have myself been speaking of 'patients'; but perhaps we should go back a step and question this first.

A patient (as opposed to an agent) is one who has something done to *her*; she is passive. In pre-industrial societies patients did not exist. In our society a patient is the raw material of the health care system. The patient is one who gives up self-control to others (experts) who are in a position to explain, predict and control her bodily functions. To be a patient is to be 'communicated with' but not talked to, to be 'manipulated' but not touched; to be a patient is to be treated as a generality, not as a unique person. Science deals in generalisations, so the unwell person is seen as a 'case', as an instance of some scientific generality. When the unwell talks to the doctor, only the distorted echo of a patient is heard. The doctor listens only to that which pertains to the objective and scientific evaluation.

The first moral error of modern health care is to conceive being unwell as primarily a biological dysfunction. Medicine, which dominates health care, presents illness as something defined objectively – the doctor or pathologist identifies it independently of the unwell person herself. Unwellness is reduced to pathology. And medicine forever extends its control, so that even such things as pregnancy, childbirth, ageing and quirks of character become objects for pathological investigation and treatment.

The interventions proposed by health care so often take away the control that the unwell need to become well, and health care instead employs its own 'superior' technical control, supposedly on the part of the unwell person in order to address the person's dysfunctional body. In doing this it characteristically adopts procedures which make it more, not less, difficult for the patient to regain control. In short, health care gains control by turning the unwell (and many of the well too) into patients, by presenting people with a new perception of themselves as objects of science and technology.

Nursing, especially hospital nursing, has always been controlled by the medical establishment, and although it claims as its own province the care of the patient, as opposed to treatment and cure, it has been profoundly influenced by the biomedical model. Without patients there would be no doctors and nurses, and without doctors and nurses there would be no patients.

An assumption of Project 2000 is that the biomedical model, and all its ramifications in practice, needs challenging and changing. Now it might appear that New Right ideology is also taking issue with the traditional conceptions, but it is not really an ally at all, for it has something quite different in mind – the consumer.

It is one thing to take issue with the social construction of patients, as I am. But it is quite another to give up patients for consumers, which I certainly would not want to do. If the unwell, and many of the well, become consumers, what do nurses become? Consumers are buyers, customers, end-users, purchasers, shoppers, clients. They are one side of an commodity exchange relation. The other side of that relation presumably are producers, sellers, providers, retailers, dealers, vendors. I would not argue that love, for example, cannot be put up for sale; although one may well wonder at the end of the transaction whether it is really love that one has purchased. I think the same goes for care. Dealers in care should not be surprised if purchasers complain that there is more to care than technical expertise. But then the purchasers should not imagine that anything more than technical expertise can be available for money.

There is, of course, another strand in the history of nursing, another conception which has had to fight for survival. In some ways Project 2000 may be regarded as trying to 'return to the source', to reconnect with a lost ideal, but in a new way. That ideal is the nurse as health carer *par excellence*, addressing the well along with the unwell, dealing with people rather than people's bodies, caring for people in the context of their families and friends, helping people to overcome certain life problems with their own judgement and understanding. For this health carer the person she cared for was never really a 'patient', and she was never really a 'nurse' as it has come to be biomedically understood. In some ways Project 2000 attempts to revivify this ideal.

Community and care

Project 2000 is premised on a shift to community care and a recognition of community-based values (see below). Again, there is a danger of misappropriation here, for the New Right too speaks of the community. But is it speaking the same language? What does the New Right ideology of family and community, with its moral authoritarianism, and patriarchal and Victorian values, mean for nursing?

It means, most importantly, that *caring* responsibilities are being taken away from nurses. There is a subtle shift taking place in the very conception of the nurse. As she loses her 'nanny' image she is taking on other images. One image is that of nurse as technician, who is there simply to back up with skilled technical support. The notion of 'role extension' often feeds into this image. Another image, less flattering, is that of nurse as shop assistant, helping the management to sell its goods in the open market.

Evidence of the shifting ideology of nursing, and the conflicting images of the nurse which are now emerging, is to be found in the crisis in health visiting, in the vagueness about the practice nurse's role, and in the tension which exists between these two professional groups. The ideology of family self-help results in less importance being attached to the preventive health care role. It is not surprising that in many areas public health is deteriorating. The Health Education Authority has recently announced that immunisation rates for children in some inner city areas (such as London, Birmingham, Newcastle) are now lower than in some developing countries. Diseases such as TB are reappearing.

If in terms of New Right ideology the health visitor is seen as an interfering nanny, the practice nurse is seen as the new GP's marketing researcher, public relations officer and senior shop assistant all rolled into one. Of course, the precise role of the practice nurse is still taking shape, and it is quite possible that she will be in a position to respond sensitively to patients' needs and act fairly autonomously in the patients' best interests. Let us hope so, for that would accord with the Project 2000 vision of the future.

However, I suspect that the role of the practice nurse cannot be separated from the New Right's market-oriented policies on general practice and its reluctance to provide resources and a coherent plan for community care.

Certainly, the NHS reforms will boost the existing trend to larger practices (and so-called 'health centres') and gradually wipe out the small practice and the GP who works on his or her own. It is tempting to ask whether the practice nurse, working for a large practice, is simply there to provide a low-cost substitute for the personal care which the doctor is now unable to give because he spends so much time at his computer spreadsheet. Such a substitution may, of course, be a good thing, but only if the education, resources and support are given to the practice nurse.

I raise this issue because it is, after all, a moral and ethical issue. The entire question of the nature of nursing in the community, whether in the guise of health visitor, midwife, practice nurse, or district nurse, needs clarification. Without this clarification Project 2000's rather abstract proposals on community-centred education will be given real flesh by New Right aims and objectives. Project 2000 certainly never meant to provide sheep's clothing for the wolf.

But there can be little doubt that the present Government policies based on the ideology of family self-help are eroding a meaningful caring role for nurses and midwives in the community.

Secrecy

The Project 2000 Report (¹) conceives the practitioner as one who can 'network' with a wide variety of individuals, institutions and agencies. It states: 'At the level of registration, the practitioner will need to be politically aware and to have had a grounding in the policy issues which surround practice.' (p. 40)

This presupposes that the political, administrative, managerial and legal environment of health care will accommodate and permit this kind of open cooperative *modus operandi*, and indeed *modus vivendi*. However, the new provider unit competitiveness is breeding a new secrecy, and a new ruthlessness on the part of employers.

It is already clear that nursing will need to put up resistance if the 'new nurse' is to prevail over the 'new manager'. This will not be easy as long as nursing remains in its presently atomised form with little sense of corporate identity and corporate objectives and interests. The very fact that 'whistle-blowing' could now become a major issue indicates that a struggle is taking place, a struggle between nurse as patient advocate and nurse as co-opted member of the Health Care Establishment – an Establishment increasingly divided between an industrial mass-production sector for the poor and a hotel services sector for the rich.

Indeed, there have already been a number of cases of concerned nurses blowing the whistle on poor standards of care. Graham Pink's case is only the most spectacular. Secrecy about the health service first became evident in the early eighties. In 1984 a conscientious citizen went to court following Brent Health Authority's exclusion of the public from a meeting held to consider cuts in health expenditure. Some members of the public had the idea that they had a right at least to attend such a meeting, and possibly to make their views known. Indeed, there is a Public Bodies (Admissions to Meetings) Act of 1960 which requires a health authority to make its meetings open to the public. The judge in the case made it quite clear that the public had no right to participate. He said: 'of course, the right is not a right to participate in anything that is going on, but merely to observe what is going on' (⁴).

95

'Confidentiality' in health care, once a concept associated with protection of the patient, has recently come to be synonymous with secrecy and the protection of health care providers. Negotiations between health authorities and medical supplies manufacturers for sponsorship are confidential, conditions of work however appalling are confidential, and Trust plans are confidential. Many of the new competitive NHS provider units, more conscious of their public reputation than of the real quality of their services, now expect nurses and other employees to sign contracts which bind them to public silence on issues of standards. Is this another way in which the New Right means to enhance patient choice?

It is not as though the Government does not understand the issue – it has consistently frustrated attempts to introduce a Freedom of Information Act. And, do the nurses and doctors of this country really have to wait for the European Court to point out to our Government that such 'gagging' contracts of employment are illegal?

If being 'politically aware' means anything nurses must be fully acquainted with the political and legal dimensions of the struggle for greater democracy and accountability in our public institutions – the demands for a Freedom of Information Act, for a Bill of Rights, for Acts to protect employees against victimisation, for a reform of the industrial tribunal system, for the indigenisation of European Community legislation, for a strengthening of the powers of Community Health Councils, for the reform of the General Medical Council and so on. The seed of Project 2000 sown on the arid ground of our contemporary undemocratic and outdated social and political life will surely shrivel and die.

The great ambivalence

In this section I will look at the moral and ethical assumptions and implications of the Project 2000 Report, and in the next section I will look at the curriculum proposals for Ethics as a taught subject. The two are connected – for the very fact that the Report attaches importance to Ethics in nurse education is itself a moral statement, and an exhortation against the decline of nursing into mere technique.

I shall now pick out three features of the Report which have special relevance to Ethics: the hospital-community balance; the creation of a cadre of 'aides' (or health care assistants); and the competencies of the new practitioner.

The new service balance

Recognising that many health authorities are planning for a shift of balance away from hospital-based services to new ones based in the community, the Project 2000 Report accepts the need for 'a reorientation of initial preparation towards the community ...' (p. 19). The Report points out that 'many in health visiting and midwifery claim that their students must 'unlearn' this hospital and disease-linked bias.' (p. 26) For example, the Report notes, and endorses, the new emphasis of official policy documents on care of mentally handicapped people: 'Individualised treatment and care plans, normalisation of daily life and support for carers are major themes – so too are respecting people's rights and choices, and keeping children in particular out of statutory care.' (p. 18).

Understood in the right spirit this could have profound moral and ethical implications. Simply by practising on the home 'territory' of clients rather than on the alienating territory of the 'authorities' (namely hospitals, with all their bureaucratic symbols, rituals and taboos) the nurse will be in a better position to recognise the values, rights and freedoms of clients. Imposing oneself on people in their own homes is not nearly so easy as it is on a ward round in a large 'Nightingale ward'.

There is new hope in the promise that hospital-style nursing, with its subservience to the Medical Establishment and its biomedical presuppositions and attitudes, will at some time in the future no longer provide the centre of gravity for health care. That centre will have shifted to the community where, we are promised, nurses will practise with greater freedom and independence, *nearer in every way* to patients and clients.

The Report is progressive and, one hopes, prescient. Certainly, if Project 2000 fails to achieve this kind of shift, resulting only in another theory-practice gap, it will not have been the fault of the statutory bodies and their advisers. But the radical change envisaged can only take place if the Government *a)* introduces the necessary legislative changes to make health authorities accountable to their communities and *b)* increases public expenditure in the new areas suggested to be important by the Report and by numerous research studies.

So far Government support has been disappointing, to say the least. Despite superficial appearances its own winding down of hospital care has little in common with the vision of those progressives who propose a shift from hospitals to community care. In fact, its understanding of 'the community' is utterly different from that of the Report's authors and advisers. However, since this disparity is not sufficiently recognised the Government has had some success in appropriating Project 2000 ideas for its own purposes.

Patient choice is conceived by the New Right as an exercise in shopping around. It ignores three dimensions of any satisfactory conception of community care, dimensions which are explicitly or tacitly recognised by Project 2000. Firstly, a person who needs health care does not need a commodity so much as a human relationship with a carer who knows how to play a part in restoring his or her control over life, a carer who has the resources and support to play that part to her full abilities. Secondly, illness and disability are only in part a matter of life-style; the ideology of self-help results in victim-blaming for conditions that are a result of social causes over which individuals have little or no control, such as unemployment, poor housing, inadequate industrial safety, polluted air and water and food, nuclear radiation hazards, and a destructive transport system. Thirdly, community carers cannot simply address sickness, they have to address health, especially the health of pregnant women, growing children and the elderly.

The New Right has no conception at all of enabling or empowering those who need health care. It thinks it is sufficient to simply pull out the safety net and then responsibility, initiative and freedom will somehow prevail. In truth, all the signs are that its policies have further disabled and disempowered.

Aides

In my view nowhere is the disparity between the vision of Project 2000 and the ideology and objectives of the New Right Government clearer than in the

Project's plan to train a new cadre of 'aides' (health care assistants). This is precisely why this plan is so controversial.

I see this as an ethical issue. If my grasp of the rationale for the creation of this cadre is correct, aides will, by executing the more simple and routine tasks, free up more time for *nursing* judgement and action. In the Project 2000 conception the aide is not *a kind* of nurse at all.

No doubt, considerations of cost, professional status and staff recruitment under the present demographic conditions were also in the minds of the authors on this matter. In other words, Project 2000 is trying to make the best of a difficult economic and manpower situation while ensuring that patients and clients get *improved* nursing care. This is perfectly concordant with the concern the authors show for patients' rights and nursing autonomy throughout the document.

The Report contains denials that the plan will take the new nurses further away from patients, giving them a supervisory role while the new non-nursing cadre do the nursing (pp. 39-40, 43). But it is not clear to me what it is that is being denied. One might readily accept that the creation of an 'army of the unqualified' supervised by hands-off nurses is not the *intention* of Project 2000. But the issue is what will be the actual *consequences* of implementing a plan under the auspices of a Government which is primarily concerned, not with improved nursing care, but the reduction of public expenditure – a reduction justified in the ideological terms of forcing citizens and families to take responsibility for their own care? In the New Right's *laissez-faire* conceptual framework nursing itself is deeply suspect, for it smacks of patronising and nannying people and undermining their initiative. If nursing is suspect, then an army of the unqualified may seem quite an attractive alternative.

Whatever the intentions of the Project 2000 plan for aides the Government may once again appropriate it and distort it to its own ends. The Report tries to reassure us that such a distortion would have ramifications which would stand 'in contravention of the UKCC Code of Professional Conduct' (p. 43). However, it is patently obvious at present that the UKCC's Code does not in the least motivate Government, Health Authorities or hospital management to change administrative structures and the law so as to enable nurses to put the Code into effect. How else does one explain the appalling treatment of Graham Pink and other health carers who have dared to voice concerns about standards? Indeed, it would not surprise me if the statutory bodies and the Government end up on a collision course, despite current appearances.

Practitioner competencies

The Project 2000 Report is underpinned by the notion of a morally responsible and ethically accountable nurse, a nurse who has broken with the unthinking subservience of the past. Unfortunately, however, there may be ambivalence at work here too. Managers and educators are reading the Report in different ways. Is it surprising that so many of the discussions about Project 2000, in political/administrative circles, have focused on its procedural, managerial, resource and cost implications in isolation from its almost revolutionary tone and vision? In these circles its spirit has gone largely unnoticed, which is a great setback because that makes it all the easier for its objectives to be twisted and impoverished by the great self-serving interests which are ever at work in modern health care delivery.

The Report links the plan for aides with the need for a new moral and ethical freedom for nurses. In its consultations the Project Group discovered that 'There was frustration that somehow the situation had arisen such that nurses were not doing nursing, but students and unqualified staff were ...' (p. 13). The authors recognise that if nurses are to nurse they cannot be shaped as supervisors who delegate, plan and monitor.

This has an ethical dimension. I would like to think that in Project 2000 ethical responsibility is not conceived merely in the narrow 'professional' terms of being thoroughly familiar with the codes, regulations and policies and following them out of fear of discipline, and out of a will to power over subordinates. Rather it is conceived, I think, in terms of moral responsibility to the patient or client. This moral responsibility can only emerge and thrive where nurses are in a 'hands-on' relation to patients and clients. Distance and unfamiliarity breed contempt.

In the Report there is a list of 'competencies' for functioning 'at the level of a registered practitioner' which includes: 'demonstrate professional accountability and commitment to continuing professional education and development', 'recognise and uphold the personal and confidential rights of patients and clients', and 'be aware of and value the concept of individual care' (pp. 40-41). At the same time the authors admit that 'It is difficult to capture the art as well as the science in the practice of nursing and midwifery in a list of competencies; we are aware of, and would wish to see strengthened, the emphasis on caring' (p. 41). This admission hints at more than professional accountability within the hierarchy, and it is unfortunate the Report does not try to get to grips with it.

I have sometimes used the words 'ethical' and 'moral' almost interchangeably (and Ethics, with a capital letter, for the subject). However, one should be careful to distinguish between moral responsibility and ethical responsibility, that is, between the ordinary obligations that people may have to one another and the specifically professional or role-bound responsibilities. The Report does not appear to recognise the possibility of conflicts between the morally responsible nurse, sensitive to the values of individual patients/clients while respecting her own, and the ethically accountable nurse – one upwardly accountable in terms of rules and principles through the hierarchy. What the profession regards as right, and what the individual nursing conscience regards as right in relation to a particular patient, may be at odds [5].

Here, then, is an echo of the same ambivalence. The danger is that Ethics, as a subject in the curriculum could come to mean professional ethics, a new disciplinary ideology, serving to legitimise a strengthened hierarchy which has integrated an elite of professional nurses.

It is important to understand what moral freedom is, and I turn to that now, before considering Ethics in the curriculum.

Moral responsibility

Since the nineteenth century the ruling idea of the nursing role has been that of the obedient handmaiden to the expert and paternal doctor. In 1917, a leading nurse, Sarah Dock, wrote:

'In my estimation obedience is the first law and the very cornerstone of good nursing. And here is the first stumbling block for the beginner. No matter how gifted she may be, she will never become a reliable nurse until she can obey without question. The first and most helpful criticism I ever received from a doctor was when he told me that I was supposed to be simply an intelligent machine for the purpose of carrying out his orders.' [6]

Hopefully, the only nurse who speaks this way nowadays is Sister Plume in her *Nursing Times* column! Still, I suspect that quite a few doctors and managers would fail to see anything amusing here. Sadly, in many ways we still live in the shadow of the 19th century ideology of nursing. The language may now be that of New Right 'efficiency' and 'cost-effectiveness', but the essential idea remains the same. The 'reliable nurse' is now the 'efficient' one, and in being efficient the nurse (and increasingly the midwife) is not expected to ask questions about goals and purposes. If she is no longer expected to 'obey orders', she is certainly expected to comply with 'management directives' and the 'terms of the contract'.

Moral responsibility means accepting and carrying the burden of judgement and decision in matters of right and wrong. It means a preparedness to accept guilt and blame for wrongful actions and for any wrong that results from one's actions. Morality, like your bus ticket, is non-transferable: I cannot do what is right *simply* by doing what another instructs me to do. Of course, I may do what another tells me *believing* it to be right, in which case I do it because it is right and not simply because I have been told to do it.

Morality is non-transferable because each of us is his or her own source of moral authority. Indeed, morality is the one source of 'authority' which is ultimately unchallengeable, and in terms of which all other authorities can be challenged. Since the 18th century Enlightenment it has become axiomatic that no organisation, party, church, professional group, government or law is immune from moral criticism. Morality is itself the set of basic values by which anything and everything may be judged.

Medical expertise may carry authority, the authority of technical and scientific knowledge; but there is no *moral* expertise. Doctors cannot morally direct or educate nurses simply by virtue of being doctors, although they often wrongly try to do so in the name of 'clinical judgement' or what is claimed to be 'medically indicated'. Exactly the same argument applies to managers, whatever economic and administrative expertise they may have. Managers may try to direct nurses, but they cannot *morally* direct them. Only if someone acts on the basis of what they believe to be right, and refuses to act when required to do what they believe is wrong, is that person morally responsible. If a nurse carries out instructions which are morally wrong, then it is not only the person who gave the instructions who is blameworthy; the nurse is too. From the moral point of view it is no defence to say 'I was only following orders'.

Now, the question is, *can* nurses exercise moral responsibility? Are they in a position to do so? Do they have the freedom to judge, decide and act on the basis of their convictions? Allow me to rewrite Sarah Dock for a moment, moving her from the year 1917 to some Golden Age after 2017 when those in need of health care, incredibly, have more power than consultants and managers:

No matter how gifted he may be, he will never become a reliable nurse until he *refuses* to obey without question. The first and most helpful criticism I ever received from a doctor was when she told me that I was *not* supposed to be simply an intelligent machine for carrying out her orders.

Is this plausible? Is Project 2000 pointing in this direction? No doubt, we would like to think so. For what moral freedom implies is more than adherence to the demands of professional ethics. It also means challenging and shaping professional ethics; it means allowing dissent and conscientious objection and, above all, it means challenging the political, managerial and administrative, and political constraints on the freedom of nurses. For we know that there are many ways, crude and subtle, in which nurses, midwives and health visitors are still thoroughly constrained in judging, deciding and acting on the basis of true conversation with, and concern for, their clients and advisees.

And it is not enough for nurses to accept their moral responsibilities as individuals. They need the political awareness as a *collective body* to bring about the economic, social and administrative changes which will allow them freely to exercise that responsibility without fear of victimisation.

Ethics in the curriculum

With this exploration of the relation between Project 2000 ideals and recommendations and the political and economic environment behind us, we can look more closely at the guidelines for curriculum development which have been formulated on Project 2000 premises. I have said enough to make the point that education is not enough, unless education is politically informed.

If the preceding analysis is correct it must surely be important to ensure that the form and content of the curriculum optimises the potential for an informed and corporate nursing challenge to the existing health care delivery structure. Ethics may provide such an opportunity. This is not to say that morality and ethics must be subservient to political ends, but rather that moral and ethical ends can only be achieved by insisting on political changes.

The framework

The guidelines on course development published by the four National Boards for Nursing, Midwifery and Health Visiting now emphasise a nursing education which actively engages the student, promoting analytical, creative and critical abilities directed to a more engaged and sensitive patient care (7). The stated intention is to break with an educational approach which treats the student as a passive and unquestioning recipient of a limited range of practical skills.

These guidelines accept the Project 2000 Report's formulation of a Common Foundation Programme which directs students away from a conception of patients as passive recipients, and towards the notion of 'clients'. The student must learn 'to respect the values and desires of the individual patient or client … The student must learn that care is not always 'doing for' or 'doing to', and that the skills do not lie solely in practical activities …' (p. 47).

The end goal of education is now the *professional* nurse, i.e. one who assumes responsibility for her actions on the basis of a well-rounded understanding

101

of their rightness and rationale. Hopefully, the goal is also, and primarily, the morally free nurse.

When the new nurses encounter physical and mental handicap, depression and confusion, disease, disability, ageing, pregnancy and childbirth they will combine a personal approach with some understanding of the social context: the economic, political and environmental; family, class, gender and race. This is meant to contrast with a nursing subservient to medicine in which nurses are pressured to regard the patient as a 'case', as a dysfunctional organism for which there are prescribed remedies which nurses merely administer at the behest of doctors.

Cross-disciplinary

Just as there is a need to break down barriers in our professional bureaucracies, and just as modern trends in science now involve cross-disciplinary models and theorising, so too Ethics provides an opportunity for cross-fertilisation. Project 2000 envisages a nurse education which not only makes students cognisant of research and new clinical techniques, but also of what is relevant in philosophy, sociology, psychology, economics and history.

Certainly there is a danger of a directionless eclecticism in this. It may be said that given the narrow and didactic nurse education of the past this is probably not something to worry about yet. Still, there is already considerable confusion, both in official documents and in nursing colleges, about the character of Nursing Ethics. It is variously spoken of as a branch of philosophy, bioethics, medical ethics, professional ethics and law, moral education or even counselling.

It is now an urgent matter to define Nursing Ethics, if we are to avoid inflicting a meaningless mishmash on students. Of course, Project 2000 is pushing ahead with hardly enough time to give thought to this matter, or to plan for the qualified teachers and resources required. The educators need to be re-educated. There is the risk that unqualified dabblers in Ethics, who have been influenced by one or two books (usually in bioethics), will relay questionable methods and ideas to the next generation of students.

I think it helpful to distinguish, on epistemological grounds, between three dimensions or perspectives – the empirical, the analytic and the prescriptive [8]. These three should be regarded as dimensions of a single concern with questions of right and wrong, good and evil, justice and injustice.

Empirical dimension

Here the emphasis is on the description and explanation of the *facts* of moral beliefs and behaviour. The social sciences, especially sociology, psychology and political science, have various methods and theories to offer in this regard, and there is a wide literature. Students and tutors should be acquainted with the empirical studies of the moral beliefs and behaviour of health care professionals, including doctors and managers, and of patients and their families.

Some of the findings of these studies surprise even experienced nurses. To give a standard example, a 1966 study of nurse-doctor relationships in the USA showed that nurses usually complied with medical orders when they knew they were substandard. Researchers arranged for a doctor to order a nurse to administer a dosage which was excessive, not on ward stock list, by telephone (against policy), with an unfamiliar voice. Twenty one out of 22 nurses complied ([9]). I would like to see nurses conduct such an experiment in the U.K. now.

There is a great need for empirical studies of the ethics of nursing in relation to power, institutional constraints, professional group dynamics, race and gender, and so on.

Analytic dimension
Here the emphasis is on the analysis of the *form of thought* adopted in health care. The approach might be described as philosophical. Observation, measurement, questionnaires, statistical techniques are *not* employed (at least not directly) in philosophy. It involves the analysis of concepts and their relations, making explicit underlying assumptions and revealing inconsistencies, incoherence and confusion.

It is not the job of a professional philosopher to describe and explain, nor to make moral judgments or prescriptions. In fact philosophy may involve a critical scrutiny of descriptions, explanations, judgments and prescriptions.

It is very much in keeping with the spirit of Project 2000 to adopt a critical, questioning attitude, even or especially towards the law, and professional codes and guidelines. Professional ethics is largely about the distinction between malpractice and standard practice; whereas most really important questions are about the nature of standard practice. Professional ethics is about what is wrong when nurses engage in malpractice and what is right when they act in accordance with established practice; whereas Ethics should also examine what may be morally wrong when nurses are engaged in established and standard practice. Only in this way is the frontier of practice pushed forward, and the paradigm of nursing changed.

Of course, philosophical scrutiny may change one's understanding of the facts presented by empirical studies, and may lead one to question the coherence, sense or wisdom of our present health care thinking and may provide a conceptual platform for new moral and ethical judgments. To give an illustration: one may analyse the assumptions in a piece of nursing research to discover that there are inconsistencies between a biomedical understanding of the patient as a dysfunctional organism, on one hand, and caring for the needy person who 'presents' for health care, on the other. One may come to the conclusion that either the biomedical model has to be abandoned or caring for the person has to be. In nursing one cannot consistently have an allegiance to both.

Prescriptive dimension
Here the emphasis is on formulating what one morally, ethically or legally *ought or ought not do*, on making judgements, approving and disapproving.

Some aspects of codes, regulations, laws, the guidelines and directives of the Department of Health, Health Authorities and Hospital Management are attempts to embody in specific rules or principles aspects of our moral life. Other aspects may work against moral considerations, or pit one moral consideration against another.

The subject of Ethics is not made up of such rules, though part of its work may be to study them. It is the inclination to conceive morality in 'professional' terms that leads to the mistaken idea that morality is essentially about principles, and can be captured in a set of principles. 'Consent' and 'confidentiality' are obvious examples of principles. Yet even a little reflection on morality shows that compassion, patience, understanding, kindness, generosity, human dignity and so on are not principles but the very ground of morality without which even principles would make no sense. It is absurd to imagine that compassion is a principle which can be taught, like respecting confidentiality. Although one may learn the principle of respect for confidentiality, one could never see why this should have any *importance* if one were lacking in basic moral attitudes, such as those mentioned.

Prescriptive Ethics may involve the identification and airing of one's moral attitudes in debate about controversial issues. Religious beliefs and tenets may enter into moral positions and arguments, and these too require recognition and discussion ([10]). It is of great value for nurses to be allowed and encouraged to recognise their moral views, for (as I think Project 2000 recognises) the institutions and practices of health care delivery have always tended to suffocate nurses as moral beings. The reader will recall my opening anecdote.

Ethics may also involve an element of moral education, although personally I am sceptical about how far moral attitudes can be instilled in the nursing college classroom if they were not already adopted gradually through upbringing. Also, there is the thorny question of indoctrination. The Ethics teacher should never pretend to be a moral expert, for there is no such thing. Still, moral debate may remind one of certain moral attitudes one has, and reinforce or weaken them.

A professional code, one should remember, aims not to resolve moral problems, but to present enforceable minimal standards of practice, allowing disciplinary action. They are reminders not resolutions. In view of what I said earlier in this chapter it should be clear that Prescriptive Ethics which puts all the emphasis on professional codes and the law, in the absence of empirical and analytic ethical studies, holds the danger of a new subservience to the professional hierarchy. Nursing Ethics, I would maintain, must be regarded as a cross-disciplinary subject which adopts all three perspectives in a coherent fashion.

Models of teaching Ethics

This is not the place to review the various models of teaching Nursing Ethics. At present, as far as I have been able to ascertain, no nursing college or department critically and self-consciously adopts any of these models. Rather, there is often a confusion of approaches, sometimes with the bioethical model predominating although, it seems to me, no one can say why it should. I mention these:

a) *A Moral Education Model*, which often draws on religious and moral tenets.

b) *A Management Model*, which adopts a counselling approach, with an emphasis on 'coping with stress', 'interpersonal communication', 'social skills', 'emotional support' and the like.

c) *A Professional Conduct Model*, which emphasises a knowledge of professional codes, Department of Health guidelines and regulations, health authority and hospital policies, accountability procedures, and relevant parts of the law. This often goes hand-in-hand with model a) ([11]).

d) *A Bioethics Model*, which adopts the philosophical standpoint of utilitarianism and/or Kantian rationalism in alliance with medical technocracy. Medical

Ethics is a narrowed down version of this model. Elsewhere, I have been very critical of this model, for it presents philosophers as moral experts who have 'reasons' which we must accept for doing this or not doing that. Often they pretend to employ metaphysical theories such as 'utilitarianism' or 'deontology' in a prescriptive way ([12]).

e) *A Clinical Ethics Model,* which focuses on resolving the moral problems which arise in the care of individual patients from the perspective of the clinician involved (doctor, not nurse), and using a casuistic method ([13]).

f) *An Engaged Ethics Model,* which takes as its point of departure a critique of contemporary health care systems and practices, and of the power and ideology which maintain them – a critique rooted in the experiences of clients and nurses ([14]).

It is the last which I would like to see adopted, and the analysis in the previous two sections of this chapter may be taken as a justification for adopting it. If one has no sense at all that there is something very wrong with our health care establishment, no sense of the patterns of thought which legitimise this wrongness, then Ethics can only provide more support for the *status quo,* more expertise, more disempowerment of patients and of all of us when we become old, sick and tired.

Ethics is not above everything; it too is divided, for it is part of the ideological struggle over the control of people's lives. Ethics which pretends to be neutral is really a defence of those already in control of others. The participants (patients, clients, nurses, midwives, doctors, managers etc.) in a situation of moral difficulty are both the sources of moral issues and the resources for resolving them (or failing to do so). Resolution, however, does not necessarily take the shape of the acceptance of good reasons, compromise or consensus.

The Queen Charlotte's model

At Queen Charlotte's College, of which the National Centre for Nursing & Midwifery Ethics is a unit, we are doing our best to *integrate* Ethics into the Project 2000 curriculum, rather than simply adding it on as 'just another course'. In keeping with the spirit of Project 2000 the idea is to bring a 'sea change' over education in the College. The new Guidelines on Course Development issued by the English National Board for Nursing, Midwifery and Health Visiting ([7]) divide the programme into Common Foundation programme and Branch programmes. The former must be organised around five themes: the patient (person), society, health, health care and nursing. There will be four Branch courses in nursing: the adult, the child, the mentally handicapped, and the mentally ill. At Queen Charlotte's we are working with the idea that these five Foundation themes and four Branches will be reflected in corresponding short Nursing Ethics modules. That is, there will be the following Ethics modules:

Common Foundation Programme	Branch Programmes
1. Persons, Patients & Ethics	1. Ethics & the Adult
2. Society & Ethics	2. Ethics & the Child
3. Health & Ethics	3. Ethics & the Mentally Ill Person
4. Health Care & Ethics	4. Ethics & the Mentally Handicapped
5. Nursing & Ethics	Person

References to basic legal considerations will be, where appropriate, included in each module. It is also planned to have a higher level Ethics course, a Law course, a Politics of Nursing course, and a module on Midwifery Ethics.

The method to be employed is interactive rather than didactic in emphasis. It is very important in Ethics to get the method right, for it must stimulate confidence and critical discussion, as Project 2000 proposes. The general form which a module will take at Queen Charlotte's is this:

a) A very brief introduction giving the *background* to a theme e.g. consent in relation to children.

b) Brief presentation of a *case* or situation. It is important to select one which is close to actual practice and which is rich in ramifications.

c) Open *discussion* of case by the class, with some non-interventionist guidance from the tutor.

d) Short uninterrupted *lecture* from the tutor, emphasising the main points, integrating the points which emerged in student discussion, and using an overhead projector or flipchart to facilitate note-taking for future reference.

e) Final *question time*. Finally, *handout* containing annotated bibliography for further reading.

Conclusion

Nursing more than ever before needs both political knowledge and moral ideals; it needs some vision of what it should be if it is to retain a distinctive identity and rationale.

Everyone could benefit from a new vision of nursing as skilled health care because we all live in a society, indeed in a world, in deep economic, political and environmental crisis in which care for the unwell, for children, for the underprivileged is absolutely necessary.

Biomedical health care has failed, indeed it was bound to fail because its task was to solve what are essentially social problems created outside its control. Worse, in creating the illusion that scientific therapy for individuals can give us health, long life and happiness it has concealed the essential political and economic nature of so many (I do not say all) of our individual problems.

Nurses start with a great advantage over the Medical Establishment, because they have a more direct and immediate grasp of the situation of the needy. If they can resist the demands of biomedical bureaucracy on the one hand and New Right consumerism on the other and define and determine their own identity as carers they could play a leading role not only in leading and transforming health care, but in leading and transforming society.

To that end, and looking beyond Project 2000, it is time nurses started to think of themselves in corporate terms. Nurses need to identify with other nurses. They need to talk to each other about nursing, its moral and political problems and solutions, its frustrations and hopes. Only if the ideals are understood in terms of the economic and political realities of our current health care system can nurses begin to think about what is practically necessary to bring those ideals to life.

Only if nurses themselves make such a beginning, is there any hope that the ideal can be brought to life.

References

1. UKCC. (1986). *Project 2000: A New Preparation for Practice*, London, UKCC.

2. UKCC. (1989). *Exercising Accountability*, London. This is an elaboration of the earlier document: UKCC, *Code of Professional Conduct for the Nurse, Midwife and Health Visitor*, 2nd. edn., London, November 1984.

3. There is a fuller discussion of the ideology of the New Right in relation to health care in my *Nursing, Patient Choice & the NHS. Reforms*, National Board for Nursing, Midwifery and Health Visiting for Northern Ireland, Occasional Paper No. 4, Belfast, October 1991. I am grateful to the Board for permission to reproduce some sections in this chapter. See also, my Patient choice and the NHS review, in the *Journal of Social Welfare Law*, No. 4, 1990, 245-255.

4. The case of Brent Health Authority is discussed in Hillyard, P. and Percy-Smith, J. (1988). *The Coercive State: The Decline of Democracy in Britain*, London, Fontana.

5. I discuss conflicts in accountability in a series of three articles in the *Nursing Standard*, 16th October 1991, 8th January 1992 and 12th February 1992.

6. Dock, S. The relation of the nurse to the doctor and the doctor to the nurse, *American Journal of Nursing*, (1917), 17, 394.

7. I have examined the guidelines of the Welsh and the English National Boards: Welsh National Board, *General Guidelines for Curriculum Development for Project 2000 Programmes*, Cardiff, August 1989, WNB 89/003; English National Board, *Project 2000 – Guidelines & Criteria for Course Development*, London, January 1989.

8. I elaborate these distinctions in Multi-faceted Ethics, *Nursing Standard*, 12th June 1991, 46-47.

9. Hofling, C.K. et al., An experimental study in nurse – doctor relationships, *The Journal of Nervous and Mental Diseases*, 171: 80 (1966), 143. Also see various psychology and sociology articles in *The Journal of Moral Education*, published by Carfax, Abingdon, U.K.

10. See, e.g., the Catholic health care ethics journal, *The Linacre Centre Report*.

11. A very useful book, although too much emphasis could be put on it, is Pyne R.H. (1992). *Professional Discipline in Nursing, Midwifery & Health Visiting*, 2nd edn., Oxford, Blackwell.

12. The seminal text is Beauchamp, T.L. and Childress, J.F. (1989). *Principles of Biomedical Ethics*, 3rd edn., New York and Oxford, Oxford University Press. Works by Raanan Gillon, John Harris, Peter Singer, Jonathan Glover and James Rachels fall into a similar mould.

13. See Jonsen, A.R., Siegler, M. and Winslade, W.J. (1986) *Clinical Ethics*, New York, Macmillan. For a lucid overview see Carl Elliott, Solving the Doctor's Dilemma, *New Scientist*, 11th January 1992, 42-43.

14. Some indications are to be found in Doyal, L. (1979). *The Political Economy of Health*, London, Pluto. Illich, I. (1976) *Limits to Medicine*, Harmondsworth, Penguin. Turner, B.S. (1987). *Medical Power and Social Knowledge*, California, Sage. Savage, J. (1987). *Nurses, Gender and Sexuality*, London, Heinemann. Zaner, R.M. (1988). *Ethics and the Clinical Encounter*, New Jersey, Prentice Hall.

6

Teaching and supervision in Project 2000

Oliver Slevin

Introduction

The advent of Project 2000: A New Preparation for Practice, in the United Kingdom has rightly been identified as a major revolutionary change in British nursing. The changes are by now well known to most nurses and I do not propose to dwell on them in any detail here. However, some aspects of the changes will have major and far-reaching implications for the planning and delivery of nurse education curricula. These are:
- the realisation of the concept of a 'knowledgeable doer', with the demand to ensure that practice is based on a body of sound, research-based knowledge;
- the need to prepare students for professional practice in a wide range of hospital and non-hospital settings and the emphasis on preparation for 'doing';
- promotion in the curriculum of a health-orientated approach to care which emphasises health promotion and prevention *as well as* care of the sick and disabled;
- the necessity, in a rapidly changing health care scenario, to educate for change, through emphasis on critical thinking, problem-solving and learning skills *as well as* current, state-of-the-art knowledge and nursing skills.

It has already been widely accepted that these new directions in curriculum elevate nurse education to a new plane. See for example the statement on standards for a Higher Education Diploma agreed jointly by the universities and the National Board for Nursing, Midwifery and Health Visiting for Northern Ireland (NBNI, 1990a), which establishes Project 2000 curricula at undergraduate study level. Indeed the United Kingdom Central Council for Nursing, Midwifery and Health Visiting (UKCC) has specified the minimum educational award for the new programmes as being at this Higher Education Diploma level. In Northern Ireland the initial stages of Project 2000 implementation have been achieved. All colleges of nursing are linked with one or other of the Northern Ireland universities. Each course is jointly validated by a university and the National Board. And all students on the new programmes have in effect commenced study for the Higher Education Diploma in Nursing.

The utopian view of major educational innovation aspires to careful planning and preparation for all eventualities. Everything is thought-out and resolved in advance. Change agents are in place, and there is adequate support and advice for all, particularly when problems arise. However, reality tends to be a little different. There is never enough time to prepare for all eventualities and in any case many of the 'eventualities' which arise have not been (and often can not be) anticipated.

The reality is that here we are, in effect functioning in the higher education sphere, with an entirely new curriculum. This undoubtedly will present us with problems in the early stages of implementation. The students are aware that the curriculum is entirely new, that different things are expected of them. They will often have heard the rumblings of foreboding, for as with all major innovations there are those flat-earthers who warn against sailing West! Project 2000 is too academic, it will never work, the new programme ignores practical nursing skills, and so on.

The teachers are no better off. There are the organisational unknowns. What will the links with higher education entail?

This is particularly acute in Northern Ireland where arrangements are already in hand for the total integration of all nurse education into the higher education sector. Teachers are concerned about terms and conditions and how well they will 'measure up' in higher education. But perhaps of more immediate concern are the issues of the new curriculum and the new demands it will place on nurse teachers, clinicians and their students. An issue of particular concern is that of self-directed learning.

The self-direction dilemma

Many nurse educators are clearly uncomfortable with the idea of 'self-directed learning'. The symptoms of this 'disease' can be quite bizarre and in one context – that of playing around with terminology – quite hilarious. In Northern Ireland I have come across such terms as 'directed self-learning' and 'teacher-induced self-direction' which are not only structurally dubious but sound slightly obscene!

The problem lies of course with the professional implications of self-direction as an educational concept. Knowles (1975) suggests that self-directed learning involves the student identifying her/his own particular learning needs, establishing goals, deciding on what learning activities to undertake, and afterwards assessing and evaluating success her/himself. The teacher's role (if any) is that of facilitating this learning. Slevin and Lavery (1991) have viewed this position in its extreme as one 'in which the student *decides* and the teacher *responds'*.

The problem is, that to the extent to which the teacher influences what is learned, the concept of self-direction is watered down. Lawson (1979) attends to this dilemma when he differentiates between student-centred teaching, in which the teacher acts as a facilitator, and 'self-education', which assumes no direction from a teacher. Janhonen (1991) takes a slightly different tack in suggesting that self-directed learning 'entails the freedom of selecting the contents of one's teaching and the methods of teaching ... the contents of the teaching should be decided upon by students in discussion with the instructor'.

The implications here could be taken as meaning that the students decide on what is taught, but the teacher then teaches it (albeit possibly on andragogic principles). Janhonen sees total self-direction or self-education as something different again, describing this as 'the experience curriculum, in which students plan all their studies themselves'.

The problem facing nurse educators centres on the need on one hand to meet statutory 'training' requirements and on the other to meet the professional 'education' demands for a 'thinking practitioner' or 'knowledgeable doer'. This can be helpfully teased out in the following statements:

(i)   Total self-direction i.e. complete freedom for the student in selecting content, methods of learning and assessing achievement is incompatible with professional education requiring statutory learning outcomes.

(ii) Total teacher direction i.e. a didactic situation in which the teacher instructs and the student passively learns is incompatible with the concept of a professional education which stresses critical thinking, problem-solving, decision-making, responsibility-taking and accountability.

(iii) A compromise model which aims at taking the mid-line between these two stances *on all occasions* is simplistic, and does not take account of teacher, student, institutional and 'nature-of-learning-materials' variables.

My own view is that self-direction (with or without teacher facilitation), teacher-direction or a simple attempt at combining the two are not viable strategies. A more realistic and meaningful way forward is a transactional learning model characterised by partnership between the student, the teacher and the clinical supervisor. Here the student is a 'negotiating partner' rather than a 'self-director'. The decision-making is shared, and so also is the responsibility. As all three major actors share decision-making and thus ownership of the curriculum, they should by definition share commitment.

The remainder of this paper explores what this transactional approach means, in terms of the three main actors identified.

The students

Towards a transactional model

It is perhaps useful to reflect briefly on the social organisation of learning in the curriculum. The idea of learning as an exclusively individual endeavour is rather limiting. In most organised programmes of learning the endeavour is in fact interpersonal and involves students and teachers. Getzels and Thelen (1972) refer to such organised social situations as social systems. They provide four definitional statements in this regard:

(i)   All social systems have certain imperative functions that are to be carried out in certain established ways. Such functions are said to become 'institutionalised' and the agencies for carrying them out may be termed 'institutions'.

(ii) The most important analytic unit of the institution is the role i.e. the 'dynamic aspects' of positions, offices etc. within an institution which defines the behaviour of role incumbents or actors.

(iii) Roles are defined in terms of role expectations. A role has certain privileges, obligations, responsibilities and powers. The expectations define for the incumbent or actor what he should and should not do while occupying the role.

(iv) Roles are complementary. They are interdependent in that each role derives its meaning from other related roles. The role of the student is thus dependent upon and prescribed by the role of the teacher, and vice-versa.

This view of the teaching-learning milieu as a social system is essentially nomothetic i.e. it is based on normative aspects of behaviour. The dimensions of the *nomothetic* social system are as presented in Figure 1.

Social System →	Institution →	Roles →	Expectations →	Institutional Goals
(Nurse education)	(The nursing college)	(Student, teacher and clinician roles)	(Learning and teaching requirements)	(Set goals i.e. prescribed learning outcomes)

Figure 1 The nomothetic model

The most common presentation of curriculum in this nomothetic model is that of handing down knowledge to those who still do not know. This is very much in line with the ideas expressed by Paulo Freire (1970) in his banking concept of education in which 'the teacher issues communiques and makes deposits which the students patiently receive, memorise and repeat'. The problem here is that all students and teachers are in reality different and tend to behave differently in different situations. This, as suggested by Knowles (1975, 1978, 1980) in his expositions on andragogy, is particularly so with adult learners, who tend to bring to their studies a critical appraisal of why they should learn something and a wish to exercise a more personal control over the learning process.

Getzels and Thelen (op. cit.) refer to an opposing idiographic interpretation of the social system which recognises the individuality of participants. They emphasise here the personality of each participant i.e. the unique and dynamic organisation of needs-dispositions within each individual. From this point of view the *idiographic* social system is as presented in Figure 2.

Social System →	Individuals →	Personalities →	Needs Dispositions →	Individual Goals
(Nurse education)	(People as persons)	(Unique orientations to act)	(Individual needs)	(Needs-related goals)

Figure 2 The idiographic model

Within this model, the stress is on the requirements of the individual, in terms of the organisation and goals of the teaching-learning programme. In essence the student leads and the teacher – rather than handing down prescribed, packaged information – facilitates the student in where he wishes to go. The model is essentially student-centred and tends toward self-directed learning while the nomothetic model tends to emphasise a teacher-centred approach.

The problem in a professional education, and the Project 2000 curriculum is no different, is conveniently conceived in terms of these two models. A curriculum which is placed within an extremely nomothetic frame is unlikely to produce change-orientated, thinking, decision taking, accountable practitioners. Yet in a curriculum within the extremely idiographic frame, whether or not the student achieves those learning outcomes required by a statute for registration is to a large extent in the lap of the Gods!

This issue has been addressed to some extent by Slevin and Lavery (1991), with the suggestion that some degree of compromise must be reached in terms of control between teacher and student. On reflection, those authors may be of the view that umbrella statements about a balance of control are of limited value. The curriculum is a dynamic event in its unfolding; in some instances learning may have to be prescribed within fairly firm parameters i.e. the nomothetic model *must* apply. In other circumstances the specific area of learning is such that the student must be creative, or reflective, or undergo personal discovery, to achieve desired goals. Such learning is dependent on an idiographic frame. Figure 3 perhaps illustrates two pertinent examples in this regard. A skill such as giving an intramuscular injection is simple, unambiguous and for safety and efficiency must be normatively prescribed. However, developing empathic skills involves much more in terms of idiographic self-exploration and insightful, experiential learning approaches. It may be suggested from this that *how* the student learns is to a large extent dependent on *what* is being learned.

The suggestion here is that there is a need for a more dynamic interplay between the nomothetic and idiographic frames. This is dependent on a number of variables including the teacher, the student the institutional goals and the nature of the specific material being learned. This is more than a simplified bringing together of the two perspectives, but a more proactive and dynamic drawing on each by the student, teacher and clinician in partnership. This is illustrated in Figure 4. It is identified here as a transactional model, as it involves

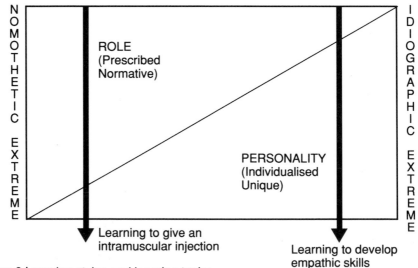

Figure 3 Learning styles and learning topics

not simply a coming together of the nomothetic and idiographic perspectives but a partnership between the teacher, student and clinician in which *both* perspectives are given consideration in *negotiating* agreed intentions and achieving learning outcomes.

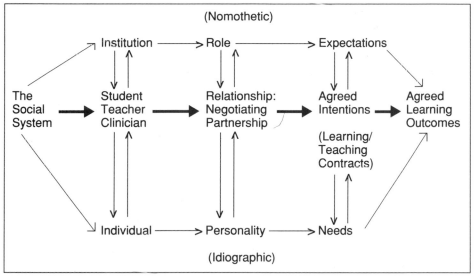

Figure 4 The transactional model

Self-direction

The implications of such a model for the student are significant. Many students may prefer the nomothetic model in which they have a clearly prescribed and passive role and in which they are lectured to, take notes, learn by rote etc. Where they are required to take responsibility for their own learning, where they have to direct this learning and are facilitated rather than talked down to by a teacher, they may feel threatened and insecure. Perhaps even more difficult may be the relationship of 'partnership' with the teacher. Many students coming from a secondary education system will find it difficult and unusual to be interacting with a teacher as a co-equal. Indeed many nurse teachers may find this equally unnerving!

The notion of self-direction envisaged as part of the transactional model described above thus involves not only having to accept a significant degree of responsibility for learning, but having to negotiate this with the teacher and clinician. It is, in effect, a partnership model rather than a self-direction model. And it views the curriculum as a negotiated order rather than a rigid 'given'.

The transactional approach, bringing together as it does the 'nomothetic role' and 'idiographic personality' of the student is particularly relevant in nurse education. We must bear in mind here that nursing is a caring activity and as such an essentially humanistic endeavour. Adhering rigidly to a normative role entails what Sartre (1957) identified as an instance of 'bad faith'. He viewed this as a state of 'nothingness', of seeing oneself as a being who merely acts out the role others have assigned to one, being nothing but what others want one to be and adhering strictly to the rules of the task. In this situation the individual adheres to behaviour prescribed by the social system and brings nothing of his/ her personal conception of morality and caring to the nursing relationship. It is the personality which brings vitality and caring to the normative role. To act out a sterile normative role is some distance away from the existential understanding of caring in nursing advocated by Oiler Boyd (1988) and others. It is perhaps what essentially has been wrong with nursing in the past. From this point of view a transactional model which takes in role-related and personality-related concerns is in fact essential in the development of a caring curriculum.

Taught practice

Perhaps the most difficult issue in negotiating learning activities relates to learning which will occur in clinical or field-placements areas and involves the student in a partnership with the clinician (usually a qualified nurse) as well as the teacher. In the past students were placed on wards under the supervision of qualified nurses who instructed them and who acted as role models. The best way to learn was on the job, working with the qualified nurse and under similar working conditions. This has traditionally been termed the apprenticeship system, and until now it is all we have known in nursing.

Students are now being faced with a new type of experience and new relationships. So too are their prospective teachers and clinical supervisors, and it can be expected that those involved will have to invest time and effort into developing these new relationships.

Whilst the precise terminology 'taught practice' is not actually used in Project 2000 (UKCC, 1986) it is used in Northern Ireland National Board curriculum requirements and guidelines when referring to that component of Common Foundation and Branch Programmes where individuals are provided with specific learning opportunities in selected clinical/field placement areas (NBNI, 1990b). The implication in the chosen title should be clear. This practical experience is a teaching-learning opportunity; it is, throughout the total programme, educationally-led.

The individual undertaking taught practice on a Project 2000 course will be a student following an educational programme rather than an employee undergoing a training. This shift and indeed the implications arising are both fundamental and significant. The UKCC states that:

> 'Placements are essential and should be planned systematically so that theory can be applied critically by the students – such placements planned solely to meet educational needs. Practical settings can be analysed for what educational experience they provide, rather than being part of a ward circuit.'
>
> UKCC, 1986

The philosophies which underpin and the methodologies associated with Project 2000 programmes in general and with the taught practice component in particular must therefore differ from those of the past. The emphasis on theory being *applied critically, by* the student, in the above quotation should not be lost.

Swaffield (1988) states that Project 2000 means a new role for the student and qualified practitioner alike and that careful consideration needs to be given to the implications of supernumerary status for supervision. Webster (1990) believes that supernumerary status is the key to removing the theory-practice gap identified in many studies of the previous system. The signals would indicate that 'taught practice' will differ from the practice placements of the past by virtue of (among other things) the different status of the learner and the fact that he/she will experience an education as opposed to a training process.

The use of the term 'apprentice' relates to the person who learns his craft on site and is entitled to instruction from a skilled practitioner/craftsman (as suggested by the Concise Oxford Dictionary). True apprenticeship training according to Beckett (1984) links theory with practice under qualified supervision. Is there a conflict then between being a supernumerary learner on an educational programme and following an apprenticeship type model?

Beckett (1984) in considering whether the terms 'supernumerary' and 'student status' were synonymous made the following interesting observation:

'Student status enhances the development of the person enabling him/her to be supernumerary to the workforce (i.e. not part of the recognised establishment figures) but not necessarily preventing membership of the team. An essential part of the learner's education is professional development demanding more than that which supernumerary status offers with its limiting opportunities.'

Beckett claims that the use of an apprenticeship model does not necessarily negate student status whereas Boylan (1982) suggests that it does.

If it were to be agreed that no conflict existed between supernumerary status and 'sitting with Nellie', providing such an arrangement was to meet learning/development needs, would this be compatible with an educational process? Here there may well be a problem. No one who has had experience of their developing practice being guided and supervised by a skilled 'master' would question the benefits obtained despite the frequent poor correlation of practice with theory. It would be recognised, however, that the teaching role of the skilled practitioner in such circumstances is very much in line with what Sweeney (1986) refers to as 'teacher-centred', with an asymmetrical power relationship between teacher and student. A particular risk here may be that students will not gain the opportunity to take responsibility for their own learning and through this develop the capacity to think critically and make decisions for themselves. They may, conversely, accept a lack of control of their learning and carry this 'learned helplessness' tendency through to their general attitudes and behaviour as qualified practitioners.

According to McClymont (1982) the concept of education differs from the concept of training and the educated should differ from the trained. She goes on to say that for one to be educated it is insufficient that one should possess a mere know-how or knack. Thinking of apprenticeship one associates this more with training than an education. Peters (1969) distinguishes between the two concepts by relating training to the learning of skills and education to the implementation of change (not really very helpful as presumably the Project 2000 nurse will require both). Peters does go on to say that education should prepare a person to be fully aware of what he is doing, why he is doing it and the implications of it. Slevin (1981) and Glaser (1971) reinforce the view that professionals who will be expected to adapt their behaviour to suit new and ever-changing situations require education not merely a training.

Clearly the *traditional* apprenticeship model does not fit. It is no longer acceptable for the job to come first, or for teaching and learning to be narrowly nursing procedure and skill-orientated. Students must learn skills of course. But in a generalisable way, on the basis of principle and in cognisance of sound research evidence where available. They must be encouraged to think critically and to develop intelligent and objective nursing practice rather than unquestioning rule-following. In this sense they are not another pair of hands. On the contrary they represent an additional demand on the teachers and clinicians who must supervise their practice. But the demand, if theory and practice are not to be once again distanced in the curriculum, is again a demand for negotiation. That is, to promote independence and shared responsibility, taught practice must also be carried forward within the transactional framework.

The teacher

Supervising

The position of the teacher in this partnership model would involve significant change. There are problems of terminology here also. While the relationship is essentially one of partnership, involving student and clinical supervisor (qualified nurse) as well as teacher, the teacher must be seen as having overall responsibility in terms of achieving curriculum ends. In this sense the teacher is the linch-pin, the co-ordinating influence. The student expects the teacher not only to teach but to give guidance and direction.

This must, as suggested earlier, be balanced against the need to promote decision-making and responsibility-taking capacity in the student. Guidance in Northern Ireland suggests achievement of this through each student having a specified teacher-supervisor or director of studies.

The literature on student supervision in nurse education is particularly scanty, as suggested in a recent paper by Slevin and Lavery (1991). However, in higher education, with a longer tradition in this area – particularly in post-graduate education – there are some useful contributions. In a study of research supervision, Phillips (1987) noted the following expectations in students:
− Students expect to be supervised
− Students expect supervisors to read their work well in advance
− Students expect their supervisors to be available when needed
− Students expect their supervisors to be friendly, open and supportive
− Students expect their supervisors to be constructively critical
− Students expect their supervisors to have a good knowledge of the subject
− Students expect their supervisors to structure the (supervision) situation so that it is relatively easy to exchange ideas
− Students expect their supervisors to have the courtesy not to conduct a telephone conversation during a tutorial
− Students expect their supervisors to have sufficient interest in their research to put more information in the students' path
− Students expect their supervisors to be sufficiently involved in their success to help them get a good job at the end of it all!

Other researchers, e.g. Welsh (1979) and Wason (1974) present similar pictures. Students in higher education clearly expect of their supervisors subject expertise, teaching excellence and a personal caring relationship. According to Welsh (op. cit.) this is a view shared by supervisors. Slevin and Lavery (1991), while recognising a counselling, pastoral aspect, advocate that the supervisory role (in the context of a teacher as director of studies) should be teaching-learning centred. This may of course beg a question in regard to the counselling needs of students.

Teaching

The capacity of the nurse teacher *as a teacher* is clearly also important. This capacity tends to be taken as given. However, Project 2000 raises some questions in this regard. Factors such as the changed status of the learner, the focus on the provision of an 'education' together with the movement to one grade of nurse teacher must have consequences for the role of the latter. Indeed, Project 2000 is quite explicit in its acknowledgement of such a change. *Nursing in the Nineties* (DHSS (NI), 1990) states that teachers should be clinically credible in the areas of practice in which they teach. *Strategy for Nursing* (DoH, 1989) asserts that teachers must be able to demonstrate at an advanced level a knowledge of theory and practice of nursing. From the point of view of Webster (1990) the issue central to the debate is the importance of teachers having clinical as well as educational credibility. Project 2000 does provide some clarification as to how clinical credibility should be reflected in the nurse teacher's role:

'... clinical credibility means serving as a role model for the student. There will be a need for much more teaching in the practice setting and this should not be left to service staff practitioners.'   UKCC, 1986

The *Project 2000 Report* (UKCC, 1986) also makes it clear that nurse teachers must be given adequate stimulation to allow them to maintain their professional expertise by continuing to practice as well as supervise. Webster (1990) claims that the 'Jack-of-all-trades' role of the nurse tutor has been a cause of 'clinical de-skilling' and the existing teachers must be provided with the encouragement and resources to regain clinical skills. Webster goes on to argue that a move to specialist teaching will be an essential prerequisite of any change. For the first time there is scope for courses of preparation to be 'education led'. But only by nurse teachers being in practice areas will best use be made of the learning opportunities available.

A significant educational argument here relates to the issue of the theory-practice gap. The problem which may arise is that the old dichotomy of nurse teacher (in the classroom) and clinician plus clinical teacher (in the wards) may be perpetuated under new titles. The building up of clinician responsibilities under titles such as mentor and preceptor and the introduction of joint appointments and lecturer-practitioners may provide an only too convenient rationale for nurse teachers to depart the clinical area. The dangers in this pattern of maintaining or even extending the theory-practice gap is very real. In this regard the work on 'theories of action' by Argyris and Schon (1974) is relevant. It will be noted that the ideas of 'espoused theory of action' (what nurses say they would do and subscribe to) and 'theory-in-use' (what they actually do in practice, which is often quite different) suggested by the latter authors bear considerable similarity to Bendall's (1973) 'correlators' and 'non-correlators'.

It would seem that for various reasons espoused or publicly proclaimed theories are not always carried through to practice. They may simply not be practicable, be too demanding or be avoided because they just do not work too well in reality. What concerns McClymont (1982) is that the action theories of teachers who do not practice are formulated away from practice and are not tested out or observed for their usefulness. Indeed they may well be incompatible with practice. Such teachers may remain unaware of the incompatability of their espoused theory with any practicable 'theory-in-use'. Students who learn action theories from such teachers may learn to pass examinations and may even be deemed competent to practice only to find that they have few usable theories of action. It is readily apparent that with teachers who possessed clinical credibility no such dichotomy would be likely to arise.

The fundamental message is simple. In any discipline, whether it be medicine, law, psychology or – as in this case – nursing, the teacher must have expertise in the subject. He/she must *know* it, be able to *apply* this knowledge to its practice, and he/she must be able to *do* it. If a nurse teacher does not *know*, can not *apply* and cannot *do* in terms of up to date practice, his/her capacity as a *nurse* teacher is at the least limited and at the worst redundant.

The Clinician

There has been considerable attention in recent years to the role of the clinical practitioner as the student's mentor. To what extent will such a concept 'fit' the new era? Mentorship as a concept, like that of andragogy had its genesis in the USA. Introduced in the business schools of American universities the idea was taken up by some American nurse educators. The term 'mentor' slipped into the folk-lore of nurse education almost unnoticed and quickly became part of the educational language of the eighties (Burnard 1990). Whilst the term may have slipped into educational language, agreement as to what the term means and the precise nature of the mentoring role has not. This has given rise to the description of the concept as a 'definition quagmire' (Hagerty 1986). This of course leads Burnard (1990) to the conclusion that if we do not have an agreed definition we cannot assume that we are all talking about the same thing. If this is the case we cannot have a unified system of mentorship training nor can we develop general policies for organising mentorship.

The problem appears to rest, to some extent, in two slightly differing and overlapping definitions. In one sense the term mentor has clear humanistic properties. For example Bracken and Davis (1989) view the mentor as someone who is 'caring', sincere, successful in their own right, unselfish, skilled and 'knowledgeable'. This is clearly a role which combines the properties of advisor or counsellor and 'significant other' or role model. Square (1987), however, emphasises a more intensive teaching role – concerned with setting objectives, providing teaching-learning experiences and regular appraisal of performance.

118

Some authors e.g. Lewis (1986) and Morle (1990) prefer to use the term preceptor for this more active learning-teaching role.

It would appear from the literature, as suggested earlier, that the main and important difference between mentorship and preceptorship is that the preceptor is more concerned with the teaching and learning aspects of the relationship, whilst the mentor, although also concerned with these things, has a closer and more personal relationship. Morle (1990) is convinced that preceptorship is a more valuable concept in nursing than mentorship and refers to the preceptor as a teaching and resource person immediately available within the clinical setting. Burnard (1990), however, still has anxieties particularly in relation to what he sees as a return to the apprenticeship style of training with the junior learning from the mistress or the master. He claims that Project 2000 set out to reform apprenticeship training and to offer instead an education to nurses. As the latter involves analysis, synthesis, creative and critical thinking he is not convinced that being under the wing of another (although he is referring to a mentor not a preceptor) is the best way to develop those skills.

There are clearly difficulties with terminology, which are a real threat to all who embark upon the definitional debate. It may be helpful, nevertheless, to attempt a crude differentiation here, as Figure 5 attempts to do. It should be stressed that this finds no general agreement in the literature, as clearly indicated above. The suggestion here is that as the new entrants progress through the

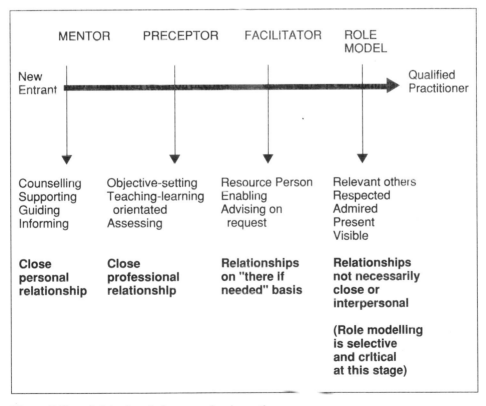

Figure 5 The clinician's role in supervised practice

early experiences, they require considerable personal support (*mentorship*) and directive teaching-learning (*preceptorship*). Later they require more space, and the clinicians role is more of a *facilitator* – providing tuition at a more advanced level, being available on request, acting as a critic and a 'stimulator' of reflection on practice. *Role-modelling* is an influence from the earliest days, when it is whole-person orientated and more affective in content. However, in the more advanced stages of the programmes it is much more cognitive and selective. At this stage the advanced learner is critically selective in relation to the nursing behaviour he/she observes, 'approves', internalises and eventually integrates. The transformation which occurs in the student results from selective *examples* of good practice rather than a single exemplar or significant other. This role-modelling influence should not be underestimated at any stage of the programmes. Using a clinical teaching effectiveness instrument, Knox and Morgan (1987) found that both students and teachers felt that 'being a good role model' and 'encourage mutual respect' were the most important properties of good clinical teachers – findings subsequently replicated by Nehring (1990).

While the sequence suggested in Figure 5 may be taken as the suggested norm, it is probably the case that the supervisor will to some extent have to move back and forward through the 'stages' in response to the individual student's needs over time.

Given the variation in the clinician's role across time, as suggested above, it may be that – as mentorship, preceptorship, facilitation and role-modelling are all important processes at given stages – a less emotive or contentious term is needed. The term clinical supervisor is perhaps more helpful and less open to misinterpretation (see, for example, Thorpe, 1979). But perhaps more importantly, the role should be seen as one in which the clinician collaborates in partnership with teacher and student in terms of her contribution.

Conclusion

This paper has attempted to address the student experience in the context of new Project 2000 courses. A central issue in new curricula will be how learning is organised and the degree of control the student will have over this learning. It is suggested that neither a teacher-centred nomothetic frame nor a student-centred idiographic or self-directed learning frame – in their most extreme forms – is appropriate. The suggestion presented here is that for the future a transactional model, in which the student is an active negotiating partner in making decisions about his/her programme of learning, is most appropriate. Although it will be recognised that a number of variables influence the curriculum, the transactional model stresses the involvement of the three main actors referred to above. This is summarised in Figure 6.

The model has as its roots the social action theories on negotiated order presented by such social scientists as Harold Garfinkel (1967) and Julian Roth (1962). It more specifically draws on Getzels and Thelen (1972) and their ideas on transactional approaches to teaching. In simple terms it *could* be suggested that the model proposes a move away from:
(a) an approach characterised by: teacher-centredness; passive students; traditional
   pedagogic teaching methodologies; little involvement of clinicians other

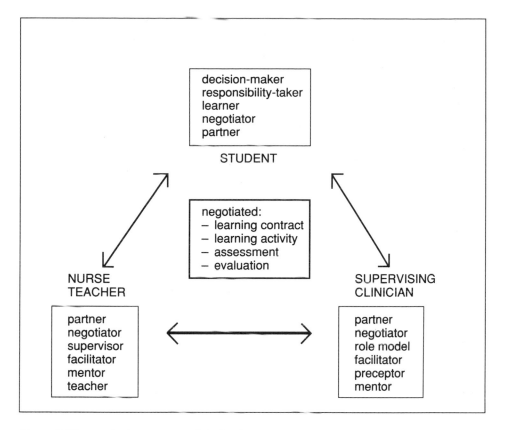

Figure 6 The curriculum as negotiated order

than in a master-apprentice situation; a wide theory-practice gap, to:

(b) an approach characterised by: partnership and negotiation; active students; andragogic teaching methodologies; active involvement of clinicians within the partnership triad in terms of all aspects of the curriculum; an integrated theory-practice approach.

This model may have a number of advantages, chief among which are:

(i) development of decision-making and responsibility-taking capacities in the student;

(ii) achievement of the normative or statutory requirements of education leading to registration, particularly with regard to learning outcomes laid down in training rules;

(iii) responsiveness to individual or personal needs and learning styles, particularly in regard to the development in the student of humanistic approaches to caring, empathic skills and moral values of relevance to nursing;

(iv) shared ownership by the three main classes of actor i.e. student, teacher and clinical supervisor, and thus commitment to a negotiated curriculum.

Like all proposals, it of course has disadvantages. The students may want to be 'spoon-fed'. It is difficult to involve clinicians when there are so many of them and when their association with particular students may be brief. Teachers, safe in the security of classroom and autocratic control of students for generations, may find it difficult to supervise studies, to negotiate the curriculum, to teach *nursing* in clinical areas. However, I see these as problems to be overcome. Given the changing health care needs of the 1990s and beyond, and the changing demands on the nurse, no one – whether they be teacher, clinician or student – can abdicate their responsibility for ensuring an effective curriculum, with patient/client care as its central concern.

The immediate future will not be a time for hiding behind outmoded, rigid behaviour or entrenched professional dispensations. There must be a dialogue between teachers, clinicians and their students about caring in nursing and how this is presented in the curriculum. The teacher and clinician must be prepared to relate to the student not only in terms of role to role, but also as person to person. This transactional relationship should not only be seen as a device for negotiating learning in the curriculum. It is an opportunity to see teaching-learning itself as dialogue. And it is an opportunity to promote in the student the future capacity to bring to bear professional *role* and personal *self* in the nurse – patient relationship.

Acknowledgement

Part of this chapter draws on an earlier paper published by the National Board for Nursing, Midwifery and Health Visiting for Northern Ireland (Sloan, J.P. and Slevin, O. D'A. (1991), *Teaching and Supervision of Student Nurses During Practice Placements* (OP/NB/2/91), Belfast, NBNI). I am grateful to the National Board and Mr J.P. Sloan for permission to draw on that paper in the preparation of this chapter.

References

Argyris, C. and Schon, D.A. (1974). *Theory into Practice: Increasing Professional Effectiveness*, San Francisco, Jossey Bass.

Beckett, C. (1984). Student status in nursing – a discussion on the status of the student and how it effects training, *Journal of Advanced Nursing*, 9, 363–374.

Bendall, E. (1975). *So You Passed, Nurse*, London, Royal College of Nursing.

Boyd, C. Oiler (1988). Phenomenology: a foundation for nursing curriculum, in *Curriculum Revolution: Mandate for Change*, New York, National League for Nursing.

Boylan, A. (1982). Responsible and accountable, *Nursing Mirror*, 154, 24–26.

Bracken, E. and Davis J. (1989). The implications of mentorship in nursing career development, *Senior Nurse*, 9, 5, 15–16.

Burnard, P. (1990). Is anyone here a mentor? *Nursing Standard*, Volume 4, Number 37.

Department of Health. (1989). *A Strategy for Nursing*, London, HMSO.

DHSS (NI). (1990). *Nursing in the Nineties: a Strategy for Nursing in Northern Ireland*, Belfast, DHSS.

Freire, P. (1970) *Pedagogy for the Oppressed*, Harmondsworth, Penguin.

Garfinkel, H. (1967). *Studies in Ethnomethodology*, Englewood Cliffs, N.J., Prentice Hall.

Getzels, J.W. and. Thelen, H.A. (1972). A conceptual framework for the study of the classroom group as a social system, in A. Morrison and D. McIntyre (Eds), *The Social Psychology of Teaching*, Harmondsworth, Penguin.

Glaser, R. (1971). *The Nature of Reinforcement*, London, Academic Press.

Hagerty, B. (1986) A second look at mentors, *Nursing Outlook*, 34, 1:16–24.

Janhonen, S. (1991). Andragogy as a didactive perspective in the attitudes of nurse instructors in Finland, *Nurse Education Today*, 11, 4, 278–283.

Knowles, M.S. (1975). *Self-directed Learning: A Guide for Learners and Teachers,*

Chicago, Follet.

Knowles, M.S. (1978). *The Adult Learner: A Neglected Species*, (2nd edition), Houston, Gulf.

Knowles, M.S. (1980). *The Modern Practice of Adult Education: From Pedagogy to Andragogy*, Chicago, Follet.

Knox, J.E. and Morgan, J. (1987). Characteristics of 'best' and 'worst' clinical teachers as perceived by university nursing faculty and students, *Journal of Advanced Nursing*, 12, 331–337.

Lawson, K.H. (1979). *Philosophical Concepts and Values in Adult Education,* Milton Keynes, Open University Press.

Lewis, K. (1986). What it takes to be a preceptor, *Canadian Nurse*, December, 18–19.

McClymont, A. (1982). *Teaching for Reality*, London, CETHV.

Morle, K.M.F. (1990). Mentorship – is it a case of the emperor's new clothes or a rose by any other name? *Nurse Education Today*, 10:1, 66–69.

NBNI. (1990). *Education Standards for the Award of a Higher Education Diploma in Nursing,* Belfast, NBNI.

NBNI. (1990). (1990). *The Common Foundation Programme in Nursing in Branch Programmes for Parts 12, 13, 14 and 15 of the Register,* NBNI/90/6, Belfast, NBNI.

Nehring, V. (1990). Nursing clinical teacher effectiveness inventory: a replication of the characteristics of 'best' and 'worst' clinical teachers as perceived by nursing faculty and students, *Journal of Advanced Nursing*, 15, 8, 934–940.

Peters, R.S. (1969). *The Concept of Education*, London, Routledge and Kegan Paul.

Phillips, E.M. (1987). What research students expect of their supervisors, *Hypnothesis*, 15, 5–10.

Roth, J. (1962). The treatment of tuberculosis as a bargaining process, in A. M. Rose (Ed) *Human Behaviour and Social Processes,* London, Routledge and Kegan Paul.

Sartre, J-P. (1957). *Being and Nothingness,* (trans. H.E. Barnes), London, Methuen.

Slevin, O.D'A. (1981). The changing role of the nurse, *Nurse Education Today*, 1, 3, 5–8.

Slevin, O.D'A. and Lavery, M.C. (1991). Self-directed learning and student supervision, *Nurse Education Today* (in press).

Swaffield, L. (1988). The new face of nursing? *Nursing Times*, 3 August, Vol 84, No 31.

Sweeney, J. (1986). Nurse education: learner-centred or teacher-centred? *Nurse Education Today*, 6, 257–262.

Thorpe, R. (1979). Supervision: is a Master's degree really necessary? *Supervisor Nurse*, January, 33 35.

UKCC. (1986). *Project 2000: A New Preparation for Practice,* London, UKCC.

Wason, P.C. (1974). Notes on the supervision of PhDs, *Bulletin of Brit. Psychol. Soc.*, 27, 25–29.

Webster, R. (1990). The role of the nurse teacher, *Senior Nurse*, Vol 10, 8 September.

Welsh, J.M. (1979). *The First Year of Post-Graduate Research Study,* Guildford, University of Surrey.

7

The student experience

Elizabeth Sweet

One of Florence Nightingale's more often used quotations is that the hospital should do the patient no harm. In the present climate of change it would be perhaps apposite that nurse education should do the student no harm.

Becker (1964) argues that in the process of growth and development two processes can be identified, those of 'situational adjustment' and 'commitment'. The former implies a response to each situation as it occurs but also implies that this response may not be consistent for each given situation. Once there is 'commitment' to the change then individual responses to given situations gain consistency. The individual can see long term objectives or goals which act as guides to decisions made, rather than responding to each situation as an isolated incident. Many nurses have made a 'situation adjustment' to Project 2000 but the real question is have they progressed to 'commitment'?

These two concepts can be used when looking both at trained nurses and Project 2000 student nurses. Student evaluations of both classroom sessions and practice experience show a considerable variation. Students attending the same placement or teaching session will evaluate the experience in totally different ways. These differences of opinion are not new. Within the sphere of nurse education, Project 2000 has highlighted the strengths of feeling associated with these varying experiences. This chapter intends to explore some of the factors which may be causing such polarity of feeling.

The macro environment (the health care services) and the micro environment (nurse education) affect both students' feelings and their perceptions about their experiences. Watson (1991) argues that many of the current changes in the NHS are political manoeuverings to change NHS working practices. As a result, nurses have been given the opportunity to raise the educational level of nurse training. Locally, the decision has been made that nursing will move into higher education, this being assisted by the requirements for Project 2000 students to provide only a 20% service contribution during their educational programme. Once the decision was made, however politically motivated, then the implementation of it was delegated, the delegation process increasing the number of people involved with no guarantee that all have the same 'commitment' to the project. 'Situational adjustment' can pervade the process of the implementation of Project 2000 with the associated inconsistency of individuals' responses.

A skeleton overview of the major changes to nursing, as viewed from the perspective of the author, can be seen by comparing Figures 1 and 2. The figures show some of the significant changes in perspective between the inception of the NHS in 1948 and the view in 1991 following the publication of the Government White Papers, *Caring for People* and *Working for Patients*. Reference is also made to Maggs' (1984) identification of the third sex, society's way of rationalising the career woman in nursing.

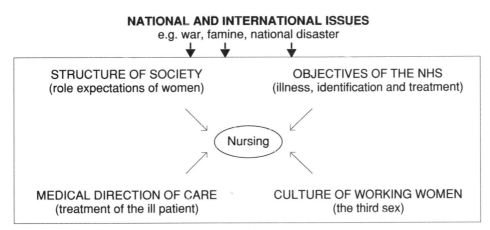

Figure 1 Nursing and health care services, 1948

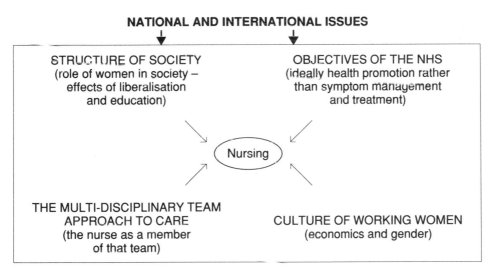

Figure 2 Nursing and health care services, 1991

If we turn to the validation process for the Project 2000 course the completion of any task should not only be judged by the end result; the process used to achieve that end result cannot be ignored and may be quite crucial to further progress. The newness of Project 2000 produced a 'situational response' amongst the validation team in my school of nursing, to the task of achieving validation of the new diploma level course. Due to deadlines, the dominant activity was towards the completion of the task, with little time or energy used to look at how the task was achieved. As a result not all staff were involved in the validation process. This has meant that during the implementation of the course, some staff have been expected to gain insight and understanding of the whole course while being responsible for the delivery of only a part. Time being of the essence, the major effort was put into delivery of the part, rather than an integration of the whole. How much difficulty this has caused teachers and students is not clear, but I feel that circumstances have been produced which have supported situational responses rather than commitment. A simplified diagrammatic representation of this is shown in Figure 3.

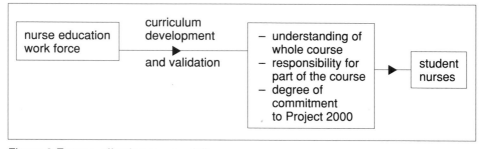

Figure 3 Factors affecting course delivery

Similar factors can be attributed to clinical staff in placement areas – the events being the implementation of the Government's White Papers and responding to the needs of Project 2000 students. The rate of the change process has supported situational response rather than commitment.

The students when entering and progressing through nurse education and working in the NHS are part of a recruitment and selection process which in turn is followed by a significant socialisation process. Failure to comply with the socialisation process usually results in total removal from the process, either not being allowed to complete the course or failure to find nursing employment. This has been summarised in Figure 4.

It can be argued that, until recently, the health care services have been viewed as secure organisations using low risk strategies to support the 'highly valued well tried solutions to problems' (Johnson and Scholes, 1989). The environment created in the 1990s moves towards, or even demands, flexible approaches, growth and development becoming more important than consensus and stability. Analysis of management structures and strategies, as demonstrated by health care journals, shows a development of organistic rather than mechanistic approaches to management. The organistic structure promotes a more rapid response to the changing demands being made on the services provided.

Nursing has been used to a strong mechanistic approach to both nursing management and perhaps even to the management of care. The move to an organistic style requires a considerable change in the culture of the organisation. The term 'organisational culture' used here is described by Johnson and Scholes (1989) and is based on the work of Schein (1985). Organisational culture is taken to mean 'the deeper level of basic assumptions and beliefs that are shared

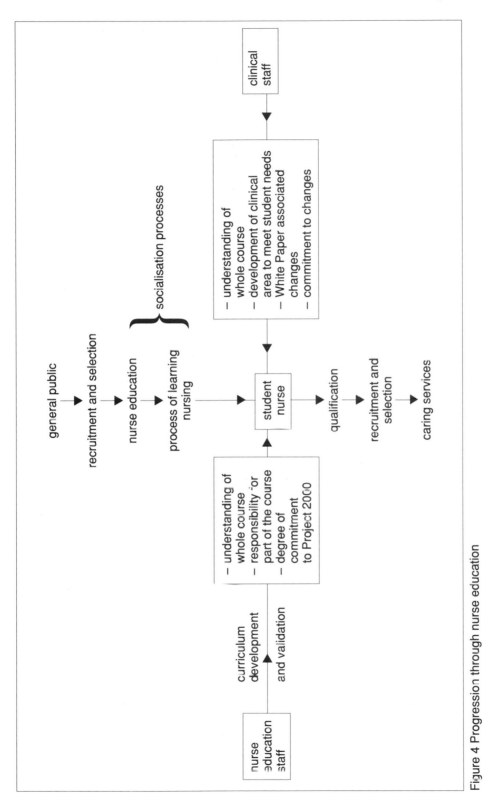

Figure 4 Progression through nurse education

by members of an organisation, that operate unconsciously and define in a basic taken for granted fashion an organisation view of itself and its environment. ... the ways (in which) members of the organisation behave towards each other, the rituals and routines of organisational life, ...' (Johnson and Scholes, 1989). Many writers on the process of change support this view of the significance of the organisational culture to the flow of change within an organisation. Student nurses are at the centre of four significant cultures as illustrated in Figure 5.

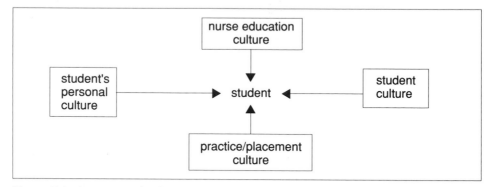

Figure 5 At the centre of cultures

The values and beliefs of each of these potentially different cultures may assist or hinder the student nurse in the process of learning nursing. It could be argued that this has always been the case, and that the implementation of Project 2000 is no different. Very simply, each of these cultures can be represented by two potentially different value systems. Nurse education may show both pre-Project 2000 rules, rituals and values and also post-Project 2000 rules, rituals and values. Practice may also present pre-white papers and post-white papers behaviour, the individuals within the nursing education system showing as a result the inconsistent responses of 'situational response' or the consistent responses of 'commitment' to the changes being implemented.

Post-placement seminars have been most enlightening for the teachers involved. The discussion of practice has given the nurse teachers insight into how the student used the placement as a learning experience and how the placement staff have responded to students throughout the practice period. Many of the placements used put considerable effort into making students feel welcome as useful, albeit temporary, members of the team in which they are placed. Students, on occasion, feel that their needs should be the centre of activity, waiting time and non-doing time being seen as time wasters. The students, at times, appear to forget that the prime concern of the practice area is to give care and that this may not always be on the student's timetable. Here it could be argued that the students are making short term 'situational adjustment' rather than looking towards the longer term goals and commitment to their education process. Figure 5 can be redrawn as follows (Figure 6) to show key elements from each of the cultures which are influencing the students' socialisation process.

The divisions within the student culture refer to experiences of the student nurses when student grants were a major issue in the press. Slogans appeared

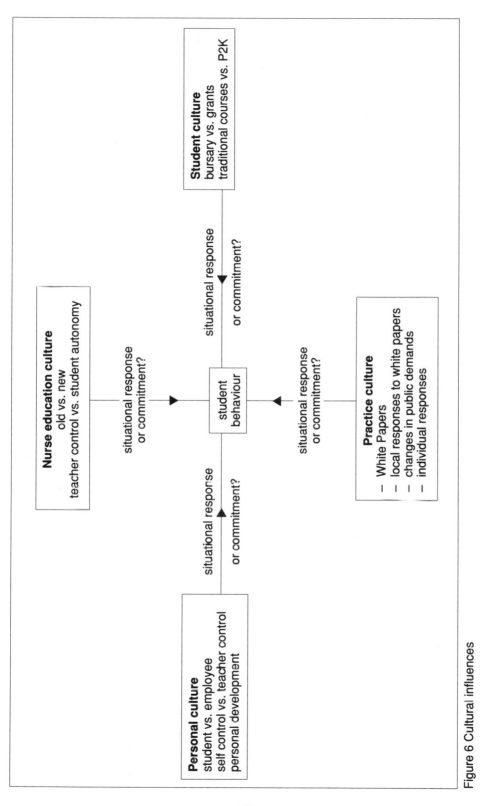

Figure 6 Cultural influences

in college denigrating the nursing students whose bursaries provided for higher payments than student grants and the controversial 'top up loans'. Looking at the implications of Figure 6 in terms of inconsistent responses shows the possibilities for mixed or confused communications between each 'camp' to be great.

An example of a 'confusion' for students was illustrated by the following situation. Students were concerned about local hospital retractions and the availability of jobs at the end of the course or perhaps they were using this as a reason to show their degree of uncertainty. Time was taken to debate the issues related to the *status quo* of nursing covering both historical and current factors. One of the teaching sessions was abandoned in order to do this since it was thought that the students would gain little until they were allowed to work through some of their discontent. The debate was informative and constructive until one student exploded by saying 'What you are really saying is that if nurses had had their act together twenty years ago nursing would be very different today.' That nurse teachers could be critical of themselves and others caused several students considerable confusion. It left the nurse teachers with the distinct feeling that some students expected them to always make the right decision! Nurse teachers being retrospectively critical of themselves and colleagues was difficult for the students to accept.

This is perhaps a reflection of a lay view of nursing with which many students enter the course. Nursing is not a profession of absolutes. There is not always a right way and a wrong way, easily identified, of nursing. The teaching strategy of encouraging students to question can easily conflict with this potentially simplistic view of nursing. Some students find difficulty in accepting the advice of teachers who refuse to say exactly how a nurse should respond to a given situation and who reply with several options for action. The student nurses reflect a lay attitude and, at least initially, prefer to be told that given A the nurse will always do B. This I have termed for my own benefit the stimulus-response approach to nursing. It has its place, *but* that place is limited and this appears to be difficult for some students to accept.

The discussion so far has perhaps indicated that this ambivalence is a destructive force. That is not the intention. Rather it is part of the process of change. Robinson (1991) argues that 'open expression of ambivalence and resistance, should not only be tolerated but also actively encouraged in order to facilitate, over time, the transition from one system of beliefs to another'. These feelings of ambivalence are part of the mechanism for coping with change. Lancaster (1982) supports the view that 'coping with change is a major personal and professional responsibility for nurses, since inability to cope inevitably reduces progress and effective functioning'. From this it is obvious in theory, if not in practice, that as nurse education is about change for students, then resistance should be responded to constructively and not destructively. Perhaps at present the latter is more frequent. Absenteeism is treated with a disciplinary approach, groups are labelled negative and difficult, teachers are labelled 'the soft touch' or 'not approachable', phrases such as 'you do fine if you do it their way' or 'management are changing their minds again'' may be heard.

Student nurses are both resilient and resourceful. Discussion with students has shown the development of some interesting coping strategies in practice areas. These strategies include active listening (even when staff are showing dissatisfaction at the changes taking place), and controlled use of questions. The students who appear to gain most from practice appear to be those who maintain the right balance between listening, questioning, offering information and participating in nursing activities. The degree of enthusiasm, however, is crucial. Over-enthusiasm can be as much a hindrance to a good clinical experience as under-enthusiasm. It is interesting to note that many of the behaviour patterns which students identify as being useful are similar to those identified by Schaefer (1991) in her article discussing the activities of clinical nurse specialists. Students do not possess the in-depth advanced levels of clinical knowledge, but motivated students appear to assist in helping the clinical staff explain what they are doing in such a way that both the student and the practitioner benefit. The good students act as catalysts to change.

It appears from my thoughts behind the above discussion and experiences with students to date that nurse teachers must find strategies for the following problems:

1 How to unfreeze students' lay perceptions of nursing.
2 How to identify the best learning strategies for students to use in areas of practice. It cannot be left to students to find this out by trial and error.
3 Having identified those strategies, how to facilitate students in acquiring the skills to use practice to its full potential while not causing any detriment to client care.
4 How to create sessions within the classroom which promote active, constructive comparison of research in nursing, theoretical concepts in nursing and the realities of nursing in the clinical setting.

This appears a lot of work for nurse teachers. Until these issues are actively addressed, the student population will retain some of its present confusion about where nursing is going and why it is going there.

1 How to unfreeze students' lay perceptions of nursing

The student learning environment is a complex mix of cultural influences, some the result of history, some the result of change. The potential dichotomy of these perspectives is not going to change; nurses today, however radical, cannot be divorced from their own history and nursing history.

How, then, may the problem of unfreezing students' lay perceptions of nursing be changed. Since nurse teachers are key agents of change, as indeed are all nursing staff in student placement areas, one answer perhaps lies in the history of each nurse, rather than in the history of nursing in general. The nurse teachers are the ones who need to address the issue of the complex mix of cultural influences on the students' total learning environment.

Shoemaker (1964) produced an interesting graded list of individuals' responses to change from innovator to laggard. In teaching the concept of change and the ideas associated with change to students I have noticed several interesting points. Firstly those students who are in favour of change in their own lives are not necessarily those who are the innovators in nursing, sometimes quite the reverse. Secondly, it is noticeable that one is not an innovator in all aspects of personal or professional life. The latter point is supported by feedback via students about the practices in many clinical areas. An area may be dynamic and proactive in one aspect of care or ward administration but highly traditional in another. For example, staff may be totally committed to using the most up to date research on pressure area care, but traditional demands for ward tidiness, exemplified by the way the openings of the pillows face, may also be demanded by the ward sister. Even in the most innovative ward there appears to be significant evidence of traditional or historical nursing practices. I am certainly not suggesting that there is anything wrong with this, merely that this is the reality of nursing practice.

Similar examples can be cited in nurse education. Many nurse teachers are extremely dynamic and innovative teachers. The didactic teaching methods were being seen less and less prior to commencement of Project 2000. Nurse teachers require time to adapt their dynamic teaching styles to the larger group numbers associated with Project 2000. However, alongside highly proactive teaching styles many of the rituals in nurse education are of a traditional nature, e.g. the calling of registers and the segregation of staff and students at lunch breaks.

It is, perhaps these contradictions which support the students' feelings of a theory-practice gap. There appears to be an assumption among some proactive nurses that the only good practice is that which is up to date and new. It may be that nurses and nurse educationalists need to explore nursing practice for what it is, activities where decisions are made under the unique pressures of a particular moment in time based on a practitioner's knowledge and personal and professional experience. Since it is unlikely that those pressures will be repeated again in exactly the same way, nurses need to remember that each decision made is a new decision, not a repeat of one made earlier. Circumstances may be similar to previous experience and decisions made then will assist decisions made now, but I feel most strongly that each decision made about client care, or staff management, is made as a result of a unique set of circumstances.

I have rationalised the theory-practice gap into a framework, so that, in analysis of the situation related by the student or observed by myself, I can identify factors belonging to each element. The framework I use sees *actual practice* as being the sum of the following elements:
- the circumstances which make a particular situation unique, i.e. different from those met before by the practitioners involved;
- reactive practice, i.e. how nurses respond to new care regimes;
- historically influenced practice due to the history of nursing;
- experience based practice, the result of the individual nurse's history;
- research-based practice as it relates to that area of practice;
- theoretically driven practice based on theories or models of nursing;
- rationalised practice as usually carried out and supported by the theoretical perspectives of behavioural and biological sciences;
- projected practice where the practitioner works with the changes in nursing theory and knowledge and becomes proactive delivering new and untried strategies of care;

Figure 7 presents an overview of the framework.

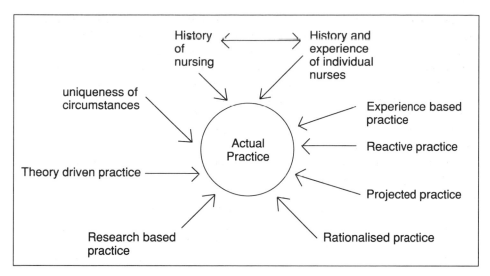

Figure 7 Actual practice

Reactive practice may be the result of changes in the direction of care or the sudden changes in patient need or new research findings. Reactive practice develops into rationalised practice which then, with effort, may become research-based practice. (see Figure 8)

Historically influenced practice relates to perceptions of nursing both for the staff and clients involved. The effect of experience should not be underestimated as a basis for safe practice. The greater the experience, the greater the confidence in the outcomes of decisions made.

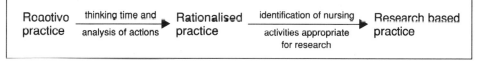

Figure 8 From reactive to research based practice

Practice is a mixture of all of these factors and there is potential for conflict between each of them. Where there is potential for conflict then there must be the potential for confusion for the students. Most nurse educationalists appear to work mainly with rationalised and research based practice – the answer guides for finals papers support this view. This may be why there is a perceived theory-practice gap, as the relevance to a given situation of historical aspects, uniqueness of circumstances and the forward thinking abilities (proactiveness) of the practitioners involved are frequently overlooked.

The process of unfreezing the students' perceptions of nursing could be facilitated if practitioners and educationalists were more aware of the factors which were directing their own practice. I am here arguing for a self-awareness perspective to be taken on the assumption that greater self-awareness will allow more in-depth analysis of one's own practice. That is, nurses, and nurse educationalists in particular, should be able to analyse their own perspective on nursing and identify which are the dominant features in which circumstances and be sufficiently comfortable with their own practice and methodology to work through this analysis with students. The work environment in which this can take place is very special. All nursing approaches should be acceptable yet also open to debate in the abstract sense, with no criticism being intended of the practitioners, a response being seen as appropriate for the standards set by that particular nurse at that particular time and under a very specific set of circumstances. This requires nurse teachers to develop a 'what might have happened if ...' approach to teaching, exploring with the students options for nursing action and discussing how slight alterations in the circumstances might have changed the nursing strategy. Criticisms of nursing action at common foundation level should also be accepted for what they are, very personal and subjective comments based on the individual's view of nursing. Objective criticism cannot be expected until students reach the branch level of theory and practice.

The environment created by nurse educationalists being aware of their own reasons for actions would enable them to identify the rites and rituals associated with each type of culture. The use of the above framework enables the expansion of the nurse education culture as shown in Figure 9.

2 How to identify the best learning strategies for students to use in areas of practice. It cannot be left to students to find this out by trial and error.

3 Having identified those strategies, how to facilitate students in acquiring the skills to use practice to its full potential while not causing any detriment to client care.

Items 2 and 3 need to be addressed but I have to admit to a personal dilemma. Nurse teachers not only need to explore the learning strategies which have proved useful to students in practice, but also how and under what circumstances these strategies have proved successful. This, I feel, can be achieved by appropriately structured post-placement seminars or structured periods of reflective practice which allow students to describe their behaviour in detail, and also allow the nurse teacher to gain a picture of potential learning strategies. The dilemma I have relates to whether I feel these strategies should be actively passed on (however this is best achieved) to all students. My own historical influences direct me to caution, simply because I have an unanswered question: can I trust all students with this knowledge? Are students professional enough to realise the ethical implications of the skills they have? I cannot answer this question at present and therefore feel reluctant to take the risk. I freely admit I am here being reactive rather than proactive on this question because I feel at present I do not know enough about student potential to be confident of the professional integrity of *all* students.

4 How to create sessions within the classroom which promote active, constructive comparison of research in nursing, theoretical concepts in nursing and the realities of nursing in the clinical setting.

The type of teaching required to analyse nursing activities is grounded in a confident and flexible teaching workforce. Open discussion of nursing and its contexts is essential. My own development of nursing ideas has been as a result

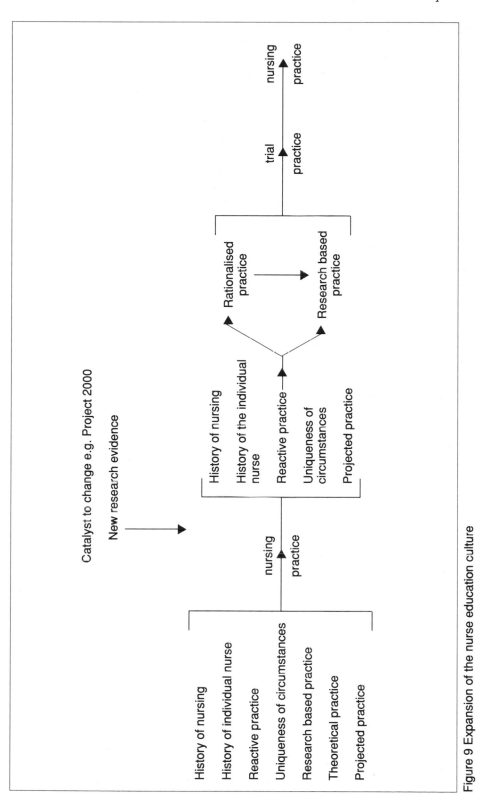

Figure 9 Expansion of the nurse education culture

of my colleagues' willingness to discuss nursing issues from many different perspectives together with caring team teaching in the classroom. Each member of staff then analyses the nursing concept being taught in the light of his/her own nursing framework. This open discussion of nursing in front of the students appears to assist the motivated individuals in creating a self development approach to nursing, accepting that nursing is more than using a nursing textbook like a cookery book. The ingredients may be the same, but each individual nurse uses a slightly different method in reaching the end product. The variance in method is the creativity required by nurses to provide for the very individual needs of patients and clients, the variance in method being due to the nurse's own model of nursing.

The environment for constructive proactive nurse education is one which allows the nurse teacher to look at:
– where nursing has come from
– where the nurse teacher and student have come from
– where they are in respect of current nursing activities
– where nursing is now
– promotion of active discussion of where nursing might be in the future.

These conditions can only develop with supportive and responsive management styles in the organisation. The people are the establishment's greatest asset. They are also nursing's greatest asset in providing the right environment for students to be the catalysts of the present, and the responsive, proactive work force of the future.

References

Becker, H. (1964). Cited by Lancaster, J. (1982). *Concepts for Advanced Nursing Practice*, London, C.V. Mosby.

Johnson, G. and Scholes, A. (1989). *Exploring Corporate Strategy*, London, Prentice Hall,

Lancaster, J. (1982). *Concepts for Advanced Nursing Practice*, London, C.V. Mosby.

Maggs, C. (1983). *The Origins of General Nursing*, London, Croom Helm.

Robinson, J. (1991). Project 2000: the role of resistance in the process of professional growth, *Journal of Advanced Nursing* Vol. 16 820-824.

Schaefer, K.M. (1991). Taking care of the caretakers: a partial explanation of clinical nurse specialist practice, *Journal of Advanced Nursing* Vol. 16 270-276.

Shoemaker, J. (1964). Cited in ENB (Ed.) *Managing change in Nurse Education*, ENB.

Watson, P. (1991). Nursing changes, *Nursing* Vol. 4 no. 43, 9.

8

Academic and organisational change

Mike Buckenham

Introduction

Much has been written on the theory and management of change within both the NHS and education. This chapter will not add to that writing. Instead the aim of this chapter is to identify the change that one particular College of Nursing went through with the introduction of Project 2000. Research into the process of change through this period is being undertaken by the National Foundation for Educational Research (NFER) and reference to their findings as published to date will be made where it helps to illuminate the text.

Change is not an easy process; much energy has to be expended in managing that change. It is also recognised that people within the change process can feel confused and anxious. That these feelings within a change are normal is recognised by Kuhlmann and Jones (1991) in their treatment of radical change, when they state that 'Whatever the conditions, circumstances or reasons for change, one cliche remains true. That is '...all change feels like a cock-up during the process of changing'. It is only with the benefit of 20:20 hindsight, supported with intelligent foresight that managers are able to accurately track their progress (hindsight) over an imperfect map (foresight).'

Nurse education has changed with the introduction of Project 2000. This is a major change. It could be argued it is the only major change that has happened to nurse education in its history. Project 2000 is not only a change in nurse education, it also affects the nursing service, and this must not be forgotten. This affect on the service however is not considered in any great detail in this chapter.

Background

Nurse education grew from the need to provide suitably qualified nurses to give care in the clinical situation, the ward in a hospital being the main focus of care, with the community seen as something to prepare for after initial training. Its organisation was therefore firmly rooted within the hospital sector of care delivery. Within this system the student nurses were employees of the hospital (or its successors) where they gained their training. Whilst efforts were made to guarantee the educational validity of the training, the needs of the service were always paramount. This focus on service was highlighted by the United Kingdom Central Council for Nurses, Midwives and Health Visitors (UKCC), in its proposals for Project 2000. (UKCC, 1986).

The Project 2000 Report made many recommendations, some of which can be traced back to Horder (1954) and which have been reaffirmed more recently in the Briggs (1972) and Judge (1975) reports. These changes have four main components. The first relates to the formation of larger training institutions with links with, or moves into, higher education. The second relates to the development of a course with a generic first part followed by a specialist second part. The third ingredient for the Project 2000 development is the move from a rather narrow hospital based training to a broader based education including both hospital and community care. Finally there is the change in status of the student of nursing from an employee of a Health Authority to a student on an educational contract receiving a bursary.

That Project 2000 was introduced seems to be linked to the enactment of the Nurses, Midwives and Health Visitors Act 1979. This led to the formation of the UKCC and the four National Boards for Nursing, Midwifery and Health Visiting which replaced the previous General Nursing Councils and the Central Midwives Board. The development of this self direction for Nurses, Midwives and Health Visitors was the impetus to look at the education required to achieve the competencies needed by the nurse as identified by the UKCC. This, linked to a change orientation in the Health Service, and the introduction of General Management with its emphasis on efficiency and effectiveness, led to a requirement of training authorities to be more responsive to manpower planning and the professional needs within the service. The scene was then set for the introduction of the project. That it was introduced with such haste within England in 1988 is unfortunate when we consider the change implications. The Government's agreement to Project 2000 going ahead with the increased costs involved was, however, welcomed by the profession. Cynics might say the approval and haste was more linked to an election than a desire to see the profession of nursing develop.

If Project 2000 is seen as a major change what is this change? Prior to Project 2000, non-graduate nurse education was organised in a similar way throughout the country. Courses were governed by syllabuses issued from the General Nursing Council. This restricted the freedom of schools of nursing in their ability to develop curricula. As stated previously the system had changed little since its inception. That is not to say that nothing had changed.

Changes had occurred to accommodate education theory, e.g. the move to a modular curriculum to help reduce the divide between 'school learning' and 'clinical learning' which was well demonstrated by Bendall (1975), but little had happened to take account of increased professional needs. The regulations governing the courses leading to registration on parts 1, 3, 5, and 8 (Registered General Nurse, Registered Mental Nurse, Registered Nurse for the Mentally Handicapped, and Registered Sick Children's Nurse), of the professional register allowed for about 28 weeks of theory within a 146 week course.

The spiral nature of the curriculum, for this was the most common organisation, meant that the student nurse was delivered a recipe of educational activity which revolved around a single level of academic achievement (Figure 1). This mitigated against the students achieving the higher levels within the learning taxonomy (e.g. Bloom, 1956). That this learning was at a lower level is highlighted by the Council for National Academic Awards (CNAA) assessment of these courses against their Credit Accumulation and Transfer Scheme (CATS). Within CATS a three year degree is worth 360 CATS points, 120 points at level 1 for the first year, 120 points at level 2 for the second year, and 120 points for the third year, of which at least 60 must be at level 3 and the remainder at level 2. Using this scheme the CNAA evaluated previous first level registered nurse training as equating to 60 points at level 1 (CNAA, 1989). The nurse registration plus Diploma in Nursing (London University) or Diploma in Professional Studies (CNAA) enabled the nurse to reach 240 CATS points, 120 each at levels 1 and 2.

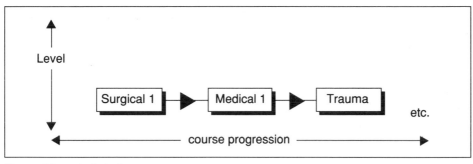

Figure 1 Level of study

The course structure, which focused on the need to provide practical work within the clinical service, and which aimed to link theory to practice, tended to the model depicted in Figure 2 . This model had the inherent disadvantage that it reinforced the fragmentation of learning and so mitigated against a holistic understanding.

THEORY	PRACTICE	THEORY	LEAVE	THEORY	PRACTICE	THEORY

etc.

Figure 2 Modular framework

A further feature already alluded to was the employee nature of the student nurse. Whilst this ensured that the student nurse was a valued member of the ward team, it worked against the prospect of systematic learning. The student, being a 'pair of hands' in a clinical environment, had to prove her/his worth. Learning, if it occurred, was therefore *ad hoc* rather than systematic.

The delivery of this training, for that is what it was called, occurred in schools of nursing which varied in size from a few hundred students to about a thousand. Some of these schools, even the larger of them, offered training for only one part of the register; for example they may have offered general nurse training but no other. Within these organisations the tendency was to organise the teaching staff in what Handy (1986) called a bureaucratic organisation (a system common in the health service).

Within these structures senior tutors, with their teaching teams, would take responsibility for a group of students in rotation. The teams provided a generic delivery of the curriculum, each team offering the full, or near full gamut of the curriculum. Variants of this would see some teachers having responsibility for a given element of the curriculum across the whole school. The advantage of this model was that it maintained the continuity of the students' learning experience and provided a clear focus for each student group.

Other schools, again using a hierarchy, were ordered on a subject specialism pattern. This form of organisation allowed specialism into the teaching but at the danger of fragmenting the learning experience for the students, and at the danger of reinforcing any compartmentalisation of learning that was inherent in a modular programme design. Due to the need to have more staff available to enable the speciality organisation it was usual to find this as a model only in the larger schools. As with the generic organisation student groups would usually be managed by a senior tutor and his/her team even though this senior tutor did not retain responsibility for the delivery of the whole curriculum to the group.

A further issue raised with regard to nurse training was the standard of education of the teachers of nursing. The profession had a large proportion of its teachers who were non-graduates, and of the graduates there was a sizeable proportion who had degrees in teaching (BEd) rather than degrees in the subjects being taught.

Nurse training was also saddled with multiple intakes of students each year. In schools which adopted a fully modularised curriculum it was not uncommon to find an intake of students commencing training every 8 to 10 weeks. This was an intake pattern driven by the service demand for a regular supply of newly qualified nurses to fill the ever present vacancies. It led to a situation which the UKCC described as 'the treadmill of nurse education' (UKCC 1986).

The college discussed within this chapter was developed from the amalgamation of two small schools of nursing and a school of midwifery. It serves two Health Authorities and is situated in a rural area of England. Courses were offered in General Nursing, Mental Health Nursing, Mental Handicap Nursing and Midwifery. Teaching was provided on three sites, one offering General Nurse Education and Midwifery Education, one offering Mental Handicap Nurse Education, and a third offering General and Mental Health Nurse Education. These sites are geographically separate, the greatest distance between sites being 24 miles.

Project 2000

Project 2000 was intended to make major changes from the above, these changes being focused on the structure and nature of the course, the frequency of intakes, and the status of the student.

The English National Board for Nursing, Midwifery and Health Visiting (ENB) publication on Project 2000 (ENB, 1989) identified that the structure and nature of the course would be different to what we had been accustomed to. Apart from the need to fulfil the European Community Directives, there were few constraints on course content. In terms of course design there was a need to have a course which was composed of two halves, a Common Foundation Programme which all students would undertake, and specialist Branch Programmes of which three of the four Branch Programme opportunities had to be offered, the Branch Programmes being: Adult Nursing, Mental Health Nursing, Mental Handicap Nursing, and Child Nursing (parts 12, 13, 14 & 15 of the Professional Register). This gave a course structure as described in Figure 3.

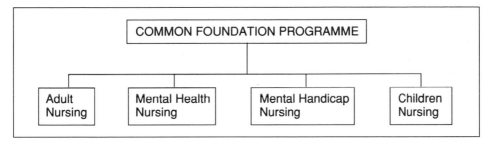

Figure 3 Project 2000: course structure

One of the purposes of Project 2000 was to change the nature of the course from a training with some vestiges of education to one of education with the required level of training. The outcomes of this new education were to prepare a 'knowledgeable doer', who could work as a first level nurse in community or hospital settings. The course was firmly tied to higher education with the requirement of the level being up to that of the second year of a three year degree programme (Diploma in Higher Education CNAA, 120 CATS points at each of levels 1 and 2), and the requirement for the course to be validated conjointly by the ENB and a higher education body (CNAA or University).

The clinical learning of the students was also changing within this new curriculum. Students were to operate as supernumerary members of the clinical teams when they went out on experience for the majority of the course. It is unfortunate that this did not extend to the full course even though the requirement remains for all clinical activity to be educationally led. This supernumerary status of the student was to enable a planning of clinical experience which was systematic and controlled to ensure the achievement of the clinical learning outcomes.

To accommodate these changes, and to get off the 'treadmill' referred to earlier, intakes to these courses were to be reduced. It was not possible to reduce to one intake per year so giving parity with other sections of higher education, but a two intake pattern was accepted. The English National Board were reluctant to accept three intakes each year although some nurse education colleges have succeeded in arguing for this option in the short term.

Finally, on the changes which have affected us, we must not ignore the change of status for the students. Student status was one of the changes considered revolutionary in Project 2000 (UKCC 1986). Students were no longer employees with a contract, rather they became students, as all other students, but with the advantage of a mandatory bursary rather than a means tested grant.

Change issues

From the foregoing it can be seen that a considerable amount of change needed to take place. To complicate matters this change was occurring against a backdrop of continuing activity where the education of students of the traditional courses (i.e. non-Project 2000) needed to be continued and supported. This change was also occurring against a backdrop of change within the National Health Service, and also a change within higher education.

Change within the NHS seems to have developed into the norm. There seems little sight of a period of stability to which staff can work. This pressure for change affected the ease with which clinical staff could adapt to the changes in student nurse education which impinged on them. It was especially acute with respect to the loss of students from the staffing of the clinical area and changing skill mix due to the replacement of the students' contribution with a mix of staff which our clinical colleagues felt did not truly reflect their needs. A further issue was the ease with which clinical staff could find time to become involved in curriculum planning, including attendance at course development team meetings so that their views on the course could be heard and they could be kept abreast of these changes.

Clinical staff in the community settings faced a different issue. Prior to this time the student experience of the community settings had been limited. With the requirements of the Project 2000 course to prepare nurses to work as a first level nurse in both community and hospital settings, the experience that students were planned to receive in the community settings greatly increased. The expectations of what students would learn during those placements also increased. Whilst the community staff supported the concept, the increased pressure of having to provide this extra experience at a time when they were undergoing change in their management organisation, and also working through skill mix changes, led to some fraught meetings between educationalists and community specialists. Through these negotiations a satisfactory solution has been found.

Change in an organisation can be considered as being either 'complex' and/or 'profound' (Kuhlmann and Jones, 1991). Complex change refers to situations where many different issues have to be addressed prior to, during and after the change. In Project 2000 this can be seen, for example, in the need to accept changes in the role of the teachers and students, changing relationships between education and clinical staff, and managing the current courses out whilst implementing the new. Profound change refers to situations where the issues need to be addressed in a different way, such as when a change in culture or values would be required. In terms of the change with Project 2000 this will refer to the change in academic values, student status etc. When change is both complex and profound it is referred to as 'radical change'. This change in nurse education is then an example of radical change.

The change issues affecting the college of nursing and midwifery which needed to be addressed can be listed as:

- new curriculum being developed and implemented
- changed academic control and validation process (quality assurance)
- changing role of the nurse teachers
- changing role of the student nurses
- developing new relationships with higher education

To complicate matters further, the change was also to happen quickly, or at least the start of the change would be rapid. Project 2000 having been approved was implemented within one year. It must be remembered that it takes three years to run out a system of nurse education so it would be three years before the total change was effected. The change would also occur against a backdrop of continued activity in all the areas the nurse education college was usually involved in. There was no extra money in the development phase to provide support to the teachers taking on the roles necessary to introduce the project so all staff would need to work harder.

The curricular design we developed went through a few changes. To satisfy the needs identified by the CNAA and the college of higher education the curriculum was moved from a spiral design which the nurse teachers knew and understood but caused confusion to our higher education colleagues, to a linear design, based on F. Greaves Curricular Model for Nursing (Greaves, 1984), which we all understood but which made vertical cohesion, the linkages between subject areas, more difficult (Figure 4). The advantage of the linear model was that individual subject areas could be clearly identified and assessed, and with an eye to credit accumulation and transfer offered the students a more favourable option if they should not succeed in the nursing course.

It was recognised early in the planning stage that this course must provide an education, which would include education in the skills needed to practice nursing, rather than being just a training course. We further agreed that this education must relate to the totality of the course and not just the 'academic'

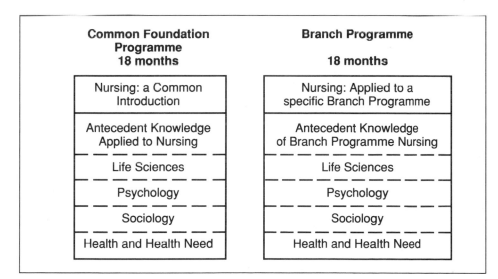

Common Foundation Programme 18 months	Branch Programme 18 months
Nursing: a Common Introduction	Nursing: Applied to a specific Branch Programme
Antecedent Knowledge Applied to Nursing	Antecedent Knowledge of Branch Programme Nursing
Life Sciences	Life Sciences
Psychology	Psychology
Sociology	Sociology
Health and Health Need	Health and Health Need

Figure 4 Linear curriculum

component. In other words the practice of nursing must be valued as much as the theory of nursing and its antecedent subject areas. The course design was therefore based on the concept that the theory of nursing underpins practice and the practice of nursing informs/drives theory. This led to the decision by this nurse education college and the collaborating college of higher education that, if a student should fail in either practice or theory then they should fail the course. There was no way that a student could obtain a Diploma in Higher Education without Registration or Registration without the Diploma in Higher Education.

The aim to provide an education also meant that we had to consider what the term 'education' meant. The view we settled on was that education meant more than the delivery of material at a higher level than previously. Education was seen as a process which involved both the delivery of the course and the experiences of the students on the course. The student experience within the informal elements of the course was seen as being of value as well as the formal elements of the course. The informal elements relate to availability of learning materials (library and audio visual aids), the access to a higher education social milieu, and the access to suitable student activities such as sport and relaxation through the student union.

As was stated earlier the new curriculum was developed over a short time period. It has been argued that curricular development should be a long term process. White and Coburn (1977) suggest that without this long term planning in curriculum development the result is likely to be a patchwork in which the design is not recognisable and where there are no safeguards against ineffectual repetitions or serious omissions. We would argue that in our development we managed to overcome most of the difficulties inherent in a rapid curriculum development. However, there were, and still are issues of the curriculum design which require further consideration before we will be satisfied with the final result.

Because of the nature of curriculum implementation we have been adjusting the curriculum in linear sequence. This has had the unfortunate effect of us never being in a situation to state categorically that what we have is what we are satisfied with. It has however, meant that most of the changes identified as being needed could be implemented before the students reached that part of the curriculum. That is not to say we have ignored any comments from the students and staff experiencing the course. As a result of such comments changes have been implemented for future groups.

It is not being argued that the process of the curriculum planning worked smoothly in all its aspects. Firstly, due to the speed of the operation it was not possible to involve all staff in all stages of the development. Curriculum development meetings were run where all teaching and clinical staff were welcome to attend. However, due to the classic time constraints we are all getting used to working under, some people were unable to attend any of them and others could only attend so infrequently that they did not feel they could effectively contribute. This speed of preparation had two other effects, firstly relating to the choice of teachers to lead in the curriculum development, and secondly in terms of the contribution from the college of higher education.

The choice of teachers to become involved in the curriculum planning was often felt to be a matter of coincidence rather than a rational choice. That is not to say we are dissatisfied with the contribution of those teachers who did the work, nor to say that we would not have used them if we had had the time to choose. Rather it reflects the fact that if we had had the opportunity to use a rational planning model to manage this change we would have identified each person's input and ensured that all those who could contribute were given sufficient opportunity to do so. Due to the need to maintain the learning experiences of our current students, and in an attempt to limit the disruption on the remainder of the nursing college activity, it tended to be those teachers who could fit the planning into their current schedules who were the most involved in the project. A knock-on effect of this is that those same teachers who had had the time to become involved in the planning of Project 2000 were the same teachers who took an early lead in its delivery and so were better placed to take on lead roles. The effect of these difficulties is well documented by Payne, Jowett and Walton (1991) who found that 'In some cases teachers felt that the choice of staff to be involved in Project 2000 curriculum planning had been arbitrary, with people falling into roles by default'.

The contributions from the staff of the college of higher education, whilst being mutually supportive of the nurse teachers presented difficulties of its own. Firstly there was the lack of knowledge about nursing in the college and so their need to quickly grasp the needs of nursing students in terms of curriculum content. This led one senior manager to comment that he felt the college of higher education had been 'highjacked' in terms of curriculum planning. There were conflicts to resolve in terms of what nursing students needed to know and what the higher education lecturers felt was required in specific subject curricula to maintain the subject coherence. A particular issue which arises here is that of when the student will be able to apply the knowledge gained with wide variations in expectations being apparent. Lecturers from the higher education college were more inclined to the opinion that there was a need to develop a base of knowledge and to develop the students' analytical skills before we could expect them to apply knowledge to practice. Nurse teachers were probably more inclined to the view that application of knowledge was a necessary process from the start of the course if the vocational development was to be achieved. In part this was probably a dilemma over the content of the message rather than a philosophical issue. We probably needed more time to examine what was being implied by the term 'apply' by these two groups of teachers each with a different history. A further dilemma was the availability of college of higher education lecturers to contribute to the curriculum planning. As with the nurse teachers all staff were already fully occupied and so found it difficult to free up time to contribute. This was especially acute when our planning stretched into the summer holiday phase.

The change in the validation process led to its own pressures on an already pressurised group of teachers and managers. The course we were developing would go to conjoint validation with the ENB and CNAA. None of the staff of the college of nursing nor the higher education institution had experience of this form of validation, although our higher education colleagues were fully aware of the CNAA validation process. Despite advice from our higher education colleagues, when the event came it was traumatic. We had expected questions on the clinical link within the course to come from the ENB; indeed the questions did come, but from the CNAA. The questions we had expected on the academic rigour of the course from the CNAA came, but from the ENB. Some of the staff were feeling devastated by the event, and all staff felt disappointed. Our submission was the first in the country to reach the final validation stage. At this point in time we were still awaiting final confirmation of the monies required to implement the project from the DoH, and the assessment schedule was not fully worked out due to difficulties in rationalising the conflicting needs of the ENB and our collaborating institution. The overall effect was that we were not fully prepared and needless to say were referred at this presentation. The experience was valuable, however, and we all learnt a great deal from undergoing the process. The next time we went forward to validation, four months later, we were prepared and achieved a five year approval.

Academic control presented its own related issues. The process used in the college of higher education was more open and also more regulated than had been our experience. The course was placed under the auspice of the Board of Business and Vocational Studies of the higher education college for its academic control to the CNAA. This means that the Course Qualifications Committee provides reports on the course activity to the Board of Business and Vocational Studies on a regular basis. As all teachers on the course (both nurse and non-nurse) are members of the Qualifications Committee, as are student representatives, service colleagues and the Dean of the Board of Business and Vocational Studies, the activity of the course is constantly open to scrutiny. Reports from the Board of Business and Vocational Studies on this course as well as all the other courses it supervises are regularly forwarded to the College Academic Standards Committee and are available to the CNAA to satisfy the quality assurance cycle of the college.

An Examinations Board also sits to monitor and regulate the examination process from the course. This board has external members who write annual reports on the standard of attainment of the students in relation to other students studying at this level, the conduct of the examination process, and on issues related to the teaching of the subjects and resourcing of the course, that can be inferred from the students achievement in the examination, to the Board of Business and Vocational Studies for onward transmission to the Academic Standards Committee. Any changes which affect the curriculum or process of examination has to be approved by the Qualifications Committee and if necessary the Examinations Board prior to going to the Board of Business and Vocational Studies for agreement and then the Academic Standards Committee for approval. This openness and regulation was a new feature for us in nurse education to come to terms with.

The nurse educators were not used to working in a system where they had to fully justify each and every curriculum decision before they could implement it. Neither were they used to working in a system which, whilst not claiming that a course document was a tablet of stone, did not accept deviations from the stated course document without the required justification and approval. We quickly learnt that it was easy to fall foul of the system unless a tight relationship between the nursing and higher education college was maintained. To assist in this relationship we developed what we termed a lead group. This group comprised, the Dean of the Board of Business and Vocational Studies, Heads of the contributing divisions, plus the Reader in Health from the college of higher education, and, from the college of nursing, the Principal and Vice Principals involved in the project. The group operated on the widest remit, that being to discuss any issue affecting the Project 2000 course or the relationships between the two institutions. The working relationships are identified in Figure 5.

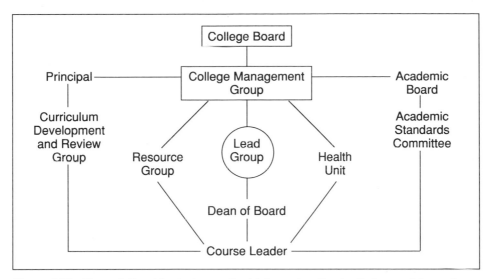

Figure 5 Working relationships between the higher education institution and the college of nursing and midwifery

The need for conjoint validation also led to consideration of how closely the nursing institution was linking with the higher education institution. We decided that due to the number of students being admitted to the course, and our geographical dispersion, it was necessary to design the delivery of the course within the campus of the higher education institution to gain the best advantages for the students. To this end we negotiated a link with the college of higher education to provide us with accommodation on their campus with full student status for the nursing students within the higher education college whilst maintaining our own identity. The nurse education institution became an associate division of the higher education institution. Articles of association were drawn up to effect this link. As a part of this association the following changes are important:

(a) the Principal of the nursing college became an Associate Head of Division of the college of higher education with equivalent rights and responsibilities of other heads of division, including the reporting relationships into the Board of Study where the Project 2000 course was situated;

(b) all teachers of the nursing college functioned as associate lecturers of the college of higher education when teaching on the Project 2000 course;

(c) the course was developed and taught by a mix of staff of the two institutions. Leadership of the areas of study being linked to ability and not to the organisation employing the person;

(d) a course leader was appointed from within the nurse education college to take management responsibility for the Project 2000 course. This person was housed on the campus of the higher education institution;

(e) payment for teaching from the higher education institution lecturers was to be based on quid pro quo rather than on financial costs. This system was the internal one operating between divisions of the college of higher education at that time.

This close attachment into higher education was seen as providing the following advantages:

Staff Resources:

The shared management responsibility for the course was seen as a reflection of shared teaching input to the new course. By encouraging the deployment of teaching staff from the two institutions with a combination of professional and higher academic qualifications and specialisms, this would offer a major enhancement in the quality of the student experience. The environment for the teaching and learning provided by the higher education setting would be matched by the context provided for the professional development in the practice areas. The opportunities created for research and consultancy, for the implementation of a staff development policy for the joint tutorial team and for increasing shared participation across a range of courses was also recognised.

Physical Resources:

The combination of the nursing college in the higher education setting provided by the higher education college offered the opportunity for the provision and development of highly appropriate educational and administrative accommodation. While the achievement of maximum benefit from the combination of library facilities, learning resources, computing services etc. of the institutions would not be immediate, the commitment existed to provide students and staff with the environment in which standards of excellence could be achieved. Well established laboratories, libraries and learning resources of all types were available and could be deployed to meet the needs of the new curriculum design. The prior experience of the higher education college in resourcing academic and professional courses in areas cognate to nurse education represented a considerable advantage.

Learning Environment:

Within the new arrangements the student nurse would combine the experience of professional development with the full range of social and cultural opportunities available to students in higher education. The environment provided by the higher education college was one in which the varied needs of students with diverse backgrounds and characteristics had been recognised and provided for. While in the first instance the opportunity for directly shared learning and the choice of modules followed in common with students and other courses would be necessarily limited, the benefits of such arrangements in the longer term were well understood. The experience of the higher education college in offering a wide ranging modular degree scheme consisting of shared academic units was perceived as a major advantage in this respect. Similarly the joint experience of encouraging independently conceived project work was one which could be developed further in the interest of students following the new course.

Validation:

The goal of achieving a student experience combining the most desirable professional development with the achievement of strong academic credentials had been central to the entire collaborative process. It was believed that conjoint validation for Registration and for the award of DipHE represented the most attractive outcome from this process for both professional and academic award for the students completing the whole course and would allow progression towards degree level and post registration qualifications in either specific or general areas. The modular provision within the College of Higher Education which includes substantial opportunity for independent study and development, was considered to offer major advantages in this respect. The joint validation would be supported by a well established procedure for monitoring, evaluating and review of the course.

Research:

With the developed links with the college and the development of the nursing college as an associate division, all facilities of the college were available to the teachers of the nursing college. The college of higher education has a research tradition in the areas of Health, Sports Sciences, Psychology and Sociology. Within these areas are many aspects of interest and value to the nurse teachers and nursing. Nurse teachers would have access to this research expertise, the ability to participate in current research projects and guidance in developing specific research protocol of their own. The aim was to develop research protocols in areas of clinical nursing and the development of nurses as a base from which to develop the delivery of the courses offered.

The organisation of the nursing college and the roles that teachers play within this organisation was also reviewed as a result of introducing Project 2000. As was previously stated this college is an amalgamation of two other schools of nursing and a school of midwifery. The amalgamation of the two nursing schools was commencing at the same time as the work on preparing for the project. This dual change of activity complicated the change issues that were ongoing.

The traditional working arrangement in both amalgamating schools of nursing was that of individual teaching teams, or teachers, managing groups of students. Within this organisation there was no clearly identifiable academic quality control system except for that operating independently within each team. To accommodate the amalgamation and introduction of Project 2000 the new college developed an organisational structure which was flattened, that is there were only three layers, and in which the teachers were organised within a matrix structure to enable the delivery of the multiple needs identified. Important roles developed in this structure were:

Course Leader – who had overall responsibility for the curriculum planning and course management of Project 2000.

Programme Leaders – one each for the Common Foundation Programme and the three Branch Programmes offered. Their responsibility was for the curriculum cohesiveness of their particular programme, especially the vertical cohesion, and to ensure effective delivery. For the Branch Programme Leaders, this also entails the curriculum of the specialist Nursing Studies Unit.

Unit Leaders – one each for the units of study, these being Nursing Studies, Health and Health Need, Life Sciences, Psychology, Sociology. Unit Leaders have responsibility for the horizontal cohesiveness of their particular units. In the initial stages of the course three unit leaders were staff of the college of nursing and two were staff of the college of higher education.

Placement Coordinator – This was a temporary but important post in the early stages of the Project 2000 development and implementation which we believed we could dispense with once the system of placements had been established. To date we still require a form of placement coordination activity to ensure the smooth running of a complex system placing students in a multitude of Health Service and non-Health Service settings.

An indication of the matrix of staff activity is presented at Figure 6. This matrix is supplemented by a staff use strategy which identifies the major teaching commitment of each teacher (Figure 7).

Function / Staff by Site	Current Course Activity	Project 2000 CFP	Branch	Placement Support	Conversion Courses	Quality Assurance
Site A T1						
T2 etc						
Site B T1						
T2 etc						
Site C etc						

Figure 6 Exemplar of the matrix structure

Teacher	Nursing	Life Sciences	Psychology	Sociology	Health and Health Need etc.
T1	9	6			
T2	9		6		
T3	6	9			
etc.					

Note: numbers in Figure 7 indicate the expected classroom commitment for the identified teacher, as can be seen this is 15 hours per week for a full time teacher. Besides these hours there is the commitment to the Personal Tutor Role, Clinical Link Role and Personal Development.

Figure 7 Exemplar of the staff use strategy

We were anxious that this new course, with its two major parts, should also be seen as one course. This was seen as being achieved through the offices of the Course Leader and through the ability of teachers to teach on both CFP and Branch Programmes. It was further ensured by the unit teams having transferability between the two major parts. This is not to say that the team remained the same for each specialist subject within each branch, but rather there remained a group of staff who maintained the academic progression of each unit.

As can be seen from Figures 6 and 7 the role of the teacher has changed. Originally teachers had a fairly standard role which had changed little over the years in that they carried responsibility for the teaching of a group of students from the start of their course to its completion. With the introduction of Project 2000 the role becomes more complex. Three factors can be identified:

(i)   being the identification of expected class contact hours;
(ii) the changing role with the introduction of specialism;
(iii) the need to develop different teaching strategies.

At a conference on Project 2000 in November 1990 I started by saying that we had a vision of nurse teachers operating within a system that allowed regularised teaching hours each week with time for research and administration (Buckenham 1990). Our aim was to establish the course in such a way that there was regularity within the timetables to allow the teachers time for preparation and self development. This was to be achieved by regulating the class contact hours to which the students were exposed. A further advantage of this arrangement was that it gave the students time for reading and reflection on the learning process they were undergoing.

The reduction in the number of intakes per year and a consequent increase in the size of intakes was one route to achieving this. One district within this organisation had been used to student intakes on a 10 week cycle, so providing a constant number of small groups of students moving through clinical experience, and a constant supply of newly qualified nurses to fill vacancies. With the introduction of Project 2000 the college moved to two intakes per year (there had been those who argued for one intake on the classic higher education model). Whilst this was fully discussed with the service managers during planning and had their full support it remains a dilemma when considering the means for maintaining vacancies for the expected outturn of students. The increase in size of groups and the consequent need to adopt different teaching styles is one of the factors which caused stress to nurse teachers within this college. It is a factor which was also identified as causing stress in the study of the implementation of Project 2000 being undertaken by the National Foundation for Educational Research (NFER papers 1, 2 and 3 published to date).

With these changes in the organisation there is a danger that teachers will feel in some ways devalued. From a position where each nurse tutor (although not each clinical teacher) had responsibility for a group of students as they progressed through their training we moved to a position where some teachers had unit leadership responsibility but most had contributing roles only. All teachers had however been involved in the personal tutor role prior to this time, and it was through this role that we attempted to achieve a feeling of responsibility for a group of students. As the number of students on the Project

2000 course increased, more teachers took on responsibility for ensuring a group of students achieved the outcomes of the course, and had access into the management of the course.

We also developed further the concept of a clinical link role to add enrichment to the teacher's role. By clinical link role we mean the responsibility of ensuring that a defined area of clinical activity which receives students is in regular contact with the nursing college and has the opportunity to discuss issues specifically affecting the experience of students in that area. It also aims to provide specific teaching of the clinical staff to ensure their understanding of the course outcomes, and that the clinical area is kept up to date in relation to changes which are happening to the course.

For the teachers this led to a situation where their responsibilities changed. For some this was a broadening of responsibility, and for others there was an increase in responsibility. For those who experienced an increase in responsibility there was a need to ensure that their authority matched their need. As already identified however, for many there was a perceived decrease in responsibility. The actual responsibilities undertaken by the teachers were very important to the future development and management of the course. As an example I will elaborate on the Unit Leader role.

Unit Leaders have responsibility for curriculum development, monitoring and delivery of their specific unit. In terms of our colleagues from higher education this was a normal role which they equated to module responsibility within a modular degree programme. This role carries many responsibilities, one important responsibility being that of monitoring those staff who are contributing to the unit, and ensuring that individual and group development needs related to the delivery of the unit are identified to management. This responsibility relates to all staff who contribute to the unit. In this organisation a grade 2 tutor as the unit leader may have as a contributing teacher a grade 4 teacher and a senior lecturer from the higher education college, both of whom would be responsible to the unit leader for their input into that unit. As would be expected, some teachers took to this like ducks to water, whilst others had difficulty in adjusting to this non-bureaucratic form of organisation. Peters (1987) discusses this concept of individual rather than bureaucratic responsibility under the guise of the world turned upside down.

To complicate matters even further this was not a 'Big Bang' change. There was no date when all teachers gave up teaching non-Project 2000 courses and took on responsibility for Project 2000 courses. The changing roles of the teachers was therefore incremental. That is not even to say that a small group of teachers were able to concentrate on Project 2000 whilst the remainder worked on current programmes. Our commitment to the current students was in some ways a hindrance to the development of the Project 2000 course. It was our intention that current course students should as far as possible maintain their contact with their course tutor, and that as many teachers as possible should be brought into the Project 2000 activity early to ease the transition.

The NFER report *'Charting the Course'* (Leonard and Jowett, 1990) relates the case of another college going down a similar route and having similar issues to resolve. The DNE of that college is quoted as saying 'the Greater Autonomy for teachers was accompanied by Greater Accountability and it proved a difficult and lengthy process to get the balance right over who decides what'. It was considered that that particular college only achieved the balance in the last 9 months of the three year programme.

Issues of 'who decides what' are central to getting this form of organisation working correctly. Yet with a multi-site and multi-activity organisation it is far from easy. The situation of the Placement Coordinator provides a useful illustration. The placement function for Project 2000 was and still remains a complex activity due to the number of non-institutional placements needed, and the number of those that are outside Health Authority control. To assist this teacher a small group of nurse teachers was identified who had a specified commitment to this activity. If due to sickness on a site the site manager felt a teacher required for placement activity could not be released for the agreed time whilst the teacher responsible for placement activity believed it was necessary to have the time agreed, who should have the authority to decide which takes priority? The site manager is fulfilling the role of ensuring that planned teaching activity for current students is taking place, whilst the placement manager is ensuring that the planning of placements for Project 2000 is on target. If the site manager is able to control the situation the placement function may be delayed causing tension between Education and Service, whilst if the placement manager is able to control the situation the site manager feels usurped in the role of ensuring the quality of education activity in that locality. For reasons such as these we moved away from the system where strict site management formed the basic arm of the management process to one where functional management prevailed. This did not remove all the tensions but rather changed the focus of these tensions.

To deliver our new curriculum meant that the role of the nurse teacher had to change from one of a generalist to that of a specialist, this specialist focus being not only in an area of nursing, but also in an area described as 'antecedent knowledge'. This specialism of role presented concern to some teachers at first as they considered it might limit their options in the future.

In the early stages of this change the effect was for some teachers to experience concerns about their involvement in this new course. There were those who were anxious to come on board with the changes and be seen to be making a full contribution to the project. For these there was the particular concern that their expertise was being undervalued or at least not fully used. Others had concerns from the opposite perspective, that is, 'Can I cope with this new breed of student who has had time to read and contemplate on the theory and practice of nursing?'' and wondered whether they would be able to cope with the questions that students might raise in the classroom or clinical setting.

This change also added focus to the need for teacher development and the need for graduate status for the nurse teachers, a situation given formal recognition in the *Strategy for Nursing* (DoH, 1989).

The final element of the changing teacher role is related to the delivery of the curriculum. All teachers of the college had been used to teaching small groups, these groups averaging about 10 students. With the introduction of Project 2000 group size increased to 75 in the first instance. This led to the need to consider teaching in larger groups. To ensure the delivery of the curriculum, including its application to the specialist nursing areas, with the staff available, and to enable the introduction of staff development within their teaching role we introduced a system of team teaching with lead lectures followed by small group tutorials as a main arm of curriculum delivery. Within our system a small group could be anything up to 20 students. For teachers who had been used to groups of 10 or fewer students as the norm this change was not welcomed with open arms. Concerns were expressed over the move to what was seen as a backward step in the education process. Larger groups are a norm, however, within higher education as is identified by Uttley et al. (1990) and it would appear average group size will continue to increase. A further concern within curriculum delivery related to whether it was necessary to have a teacher representing each nursing speciality at each session to ensure that all perspectives were covered. We cannot forget that the teachers were also having to deliver a course never delivered before at a level of teaching they had not delivered at before. To assist in resolving these matter we enlisted the help of a local polytechnic, which had a nursing department, to run a short series of workshops on delivering nurse education in a higher education setting.

Students on this course also had a change of status. What student status should mean vexed the staff of the nursing college for some time. Questions raised included: Does student status mean students need not attend lectures and other learning opportunities if they do not want to? Does it mean students can lounge around in class and not pay attention to what the teacher is saying? Can students go to the students union bar at lunchtime and come back to class the worse for wear from alcohol? Obviously students must attend clinical experiences, but if we meant what we said in our curriculum – theoretical learning underpins clinical learning, and clinical learning informs or drives theoretical learning – then if students missed either theory or practice they were not getting the benefit of the education opportunity and so the quality of future clinical practice could not be guaranteed. We fluctuated from a *laissez faire* system to an over regimentation prior to adopting a stance which we believe maintains control without being over-intrusive, and one which the majority of teachers and students accept as necessary. Students will attend practice unless there are valid extenuating circumstances. Students will attend theory unless the specialist teacher excuses them. To ensure students do attend a register of attendance is kept.

Some may ask where is the student status within this? It is our view that student status relates to the opportunity to learn. This opportunity includes learning what honouring a commitment means. As students on this course they have a learning contract which requires us to offer them the opportunity to learn and requires the students to avail themselves of that opportunity.

Allowing people to opt out of a contract for no good reason is seen as immature behaviour and as such not a part of the adult behaviour which is a part of the students' development process.

Summary

This chapter is an attempt to relate the issues experienced by one college of nursing in the implementation of Project 2000. The information is based on action learning rather than research. Each college entering Project 2000 will experience its own concerns and tackle them from its own perspective. It is unlikely however that none of the issues facing this college will face others.

It has not been an easy time. Some staff have moved through the transition with ease and are committed to their future within the college and its new course. A small number of staff have felt alienated and confused by what has happened. Some of the difficulties have been caused due to management style within the college, and some to issues such as the speed of the change required.

Other authors have reported on the changes occurring with the introduction of Project 2000. One report identified problems relating to 'communication structures, organisational cultures, course delivery systems, professional roles and identity and systems of preparation' in the implementation of Project 2000 (Robinson, 1991). Jowett, Walton & Payne (1992) identify similar issues relating to the six demonstration colleges being researched by the National Foundation for Educational Research. Colleges which are still to implement Project 2000 have had more time to prepare themselves and their collaborating clinical areas for the introduction of this radical change. It is to be hoped that the experiences of the first colleges through the system will be of value in ensuring that these colleges have a smoother ride.

Regardless of the rough ride that we have had, the staff of this college have developed substantially over the past couple of years. They can now hold their own in any nurse education or higher education setting.

References

Bendall, E. (1975). *So You Passed Nurse*, London, Royal College of Nursing.

Bloom, A. (1956). *Taxonomy of Educational Objectives*, California, Fearon.

Briggs Report (1972). *Report of the Committee on Nursing*, London, HMSO (Cmnd. 115).

Buckenham, M.A. (1990). Academic and organisational change. Paper presented at From Vision to Reality: Sharing the Experiences of Three Project 2000 Schools.

CNNA. (1989). *Academic Credit for Professional Qualifications in Nursing, Midwifery and Health Visiting*, London, CNAA.

Department of Health. (1989). *A Strategy for Nursing*, London, DoH.

Greaves, F. (1984). *Nurse Education and the Curriculum Theory*, London, Croom Helm..

Handy, C (1986). *Understanding Organisations*, Harmondsworth, Penguin.

Horder Report (1942). *The Nursing Reconstruction Committe Report*, London, RCN.

Jowett, S. Walton, I. and Payne, S. (1991). *The NFER Project 2000 Research:*, Slough, NFER.

Judge Report (1985). *The Education of Nurses: A New Dispensation*. London, RCN.

Kuhlmann, S. and Jones, M. (1991). *Managing Radical Change*. M.H.N.A.

Leonard, A. and Jowett, S. (1990). *The NFER Project 2000 Research: Charting the Course*, Slough, National Foundation for Educational Research.

Peters, T. (1987). *Thriving on Chaos: Handbook for a Management Revolution*, Suffolk, Pan Books.

Robinson, J. , (1991) *The First Year: Experiences of a Project 2000 Demonstration District*, Suffolk, The Suffolk and Great Yarmouth College of Nursing and Midwifery.

UKCC. (1986). *Project 2000: A New Preparation for Practice*, London, UKCC.

Uttley, A. (1990) Staff-student ratio set to worsen, *Times Higher Education Supplement* 941, 16 November.

White, M. and Coburn, D. (1977). The trials, tribulations and triumphs of curriculum change, *Nursing Outlook*, October, 644-9.

9

Delivering the goods:
resource management for Project 2000

Philip Cheung

Education versus resources

Performance

In recent years, the phrase 'value for money' has emerged in the educational scene. For example, in 1985, the Audit Commission for Local Authorities in England and Wales published a report, *Obtaining Better Value from Further Education* (Audit Commission, 1985); the Joint Committee of Vice-Chancellors and Principals produced its statements on *Performance Indicators* (CVCP, 1986, 1987). The Council for National Academic Awards (CNAA) publication *Towards an Educational Audit* was concerned with measurement of performance in higher education institutions (CNAA, 1989). Linked with the idea of performance indicators is the question of resource allocation for the whole educational system (Sizer, 1982). The formula used for resource allocation in higher education is now linked with performance indicators, e.g. student numbers, retention rates, the level of examination successes, the amount of research monies which institutions are able to raise.

Many may be sceptical about this system of determining funding allocation. But performance indicators do offer an overall impression of how well the organisation manages its educational business. It could be seen as a form of incentive which encourages institutions to do better than hitherto or to investigate the cause of deficiency. My concern is whether performance indicators can measure the qualitative aspect of education. The quantitative performance indicators of an educational establishment may not have any correlation with the process of education. For example, low wastage rate may well be linked with the determination of highly motivated students who will thrive in a prestigious academic environment with little assistance from lecturers. Therefore, an institution relying on its tradition may be over funded at the expense of other less well known and less well established institutions.

Resources

The validation of a course may depend on the availability of resources and resource management as well as on the actual course content. Students, who are consumers of education, focus on resources at different levels and in a different light. For example, as an external examiner for a full time Certificate in Education course, during the period between 1987–1990, I heard many students express dissatisfaction about the level of library provision, the number of tutorials and lectures being cancelled due to staff shortages, the disorganisation of the 'recall' days. On the other hand, academic staff perceived some of the complaints raised by the students as correlated with the way in which resources were managed by the institution. One common criticism is that, increasingly, academic staff are having to spend their own time on administrative and clerical duties which can be more effectively and efficiently carried out by an office manager or a typist.

There are other non-human resource factors, such as supportive services or accommodation, which can equally affect learning and the level of performance achieved by both students and academic staff. For example, inadequate teaching accommodation can be time wasting as well as frustrating to both students and academic staff. However, often the real cost to both students and staff due to shortage of teaching accommodation and other non-human resources cannot be adequately quantified and its impact on the quality of the curriculum is not revealed in the performance indicators.

Many of these issues are highly relevant to nurse education. However, unique to nurse education, is the problem of manpower associated with the management of an apprenticeship type training where student nurses were relied upon to carry out many of the nursing tasks in hospital wards and departments. Those who have been involved in nurse education will remember the unenviable task of allocating student nurses to wards and departments under the guise of clinical placement and the dialogues with nurse managers about 'even-flow' and 'peaks and troughs'. In the Project 2000 era, the human resource factor, although on the surface appearing less significant than previously, as student nurses have now been given supernumerary status, nonetheless affects the speed at which the whole educational reform can be implemented across the whole of the United Kingdom.

Project 2000 – a question of resourcing

Project 2000 is a major educational initiative in the field of nursing. How successful the whole thing will turn out to be depends to a significant degree on the level of funding. The press release of the Royal College of Nursing in January 1992 reflects this concern. The Director of Education at the RCN said:

> The extra funding from the Department of Health will help greatly to keep the implementation of Project 2000 on course. However, our concern is that the new money will be spread too thinly over so many competing needs.
>
> RCN, 1992

The competing demands are numerous. Education although important might be put onto the 'back burner'. Currently, 38 per cent of nurse education centres still have no firm date for introduction of Project 2000. This means that student nurses in those centres are being unfairly treated. At the micro level, resources are being competed for within colleges of nursing and midwifery, e.g. number of teaching staff versus number of librarians, administrative and clerical staffing levels, the amount of money for upgrading libraries, etc. The general approach to many of these resource questions is that, all things being equal, we will get what we are prepared to pay for. If we are prepared to invest more, then the dividends will be greater for the future. Investment must be made to enable student nurses to learn in an atmosphere where their minds and bodies are so cultivated that they become enlightened members of the nursing profession. Education is expensive, but the benefit is enormous. Perhaps the proverb below will signify the prime business of education:

> 'If you give a man a fish,
> He will eat a single meal.
> If you teach a man to fish,
> He will eat all his life.'

In my view, the prime business of education is concerned with the promotion of enlightenment. As Kant says 'man can only become man by education' (Kant, cited by Sullivan, 1989 p. 288). Education consumes resources and in the case of nurse education, its quality should not be compromised by students having to contribute to service provision as part of the workforce.

One of the exciting features about Project 2000 from the educationalist point of view is that nursing students will have the freedom of being students similar to those in universities or polytechnics. Yet, why are some nurse educators and nurse managers repeating the same mistake which has hampered nurse education for a century? What is the purpose for having two or three intakes a year? If some colleges of nursing in England and Northern Ireland can do away with this practice, what factors prevent other colleges from implementing such an ideal? The objections to one cohort of students a year may be related to some of the practical questions posed by service managers. These are:

– How will the wards be staffed without the students?
– What is the replacement value of student nurses? Is it one student to one qualified nurse?
– How many qualified nurses and nursing auxiliaries (or health care assistants) must be employed to replace the number of student nurses which the wards or department have previously been allocated?
– How much pump priming funding is there to implement the scheme?
– How many clinical supervisors or mentors are required to supervise the new type of student nurses?
– How much student/trained nurse contact is required?

These are important resource issues which require resolution at various stages of planning and implementation. One of the problems is that there is little data available to help us to make sense of the questions asked.

What is a dynamic curriculum?

As a profession, we have been given a great opportunity to develop and implement a new educational strategy. How does the new product – the Project

2000 curriculum look? How can the new curriculum be delivered to the students?

The practice of nursing is a divergent form of activity as the practitioner is required to demonstrate a range of knowledge and skills when dealing with his or her client. For example, a nurse is required to have:
- an in-depth knowledge of the concept of health and ill-health;
- the skills of using appropriate remedies to induce health;
- the skills of communicating with a wide range of client groups;
- the ability to exercise observational skills and the skilful application of the information gained;
- the ability to explore different methods of doing things.

What type of curriculum will enable students to gain these skills and abilities which are the corner stones of nursing practice? Stenhouse for example said:

> where a curriculum area is in a divergent, rather than in a convergent field i.e. where there is no simple correct or incorrect outcome, but rather an emphasis on the individual responses and judgements of the students, the case for an inquiry-based approach is at its strongest.   Stenhouse, 1975 p.30

The principal pedagogical aims of the curriculum are stated in *In Man: A Course of Study* (1970) as follows:
1. To initiate and develop in youngsters a process of question-posing (the inquiry method)
2. To teach a research methodology where children can look for information to answer questions they have raised and use the framework developed in the course and apply it to new areas
3. To help youngsters develop the ability to use a variety of first-hand sources as evidence from which to develop hypotheses and draw conclusions
4. To conduct classroom discussions in which youngsters learn to listen to others as well as to express their own views
5. To legitimise the search; that is, to give sanction and support to open-ended discussions where definitive answers to many questions are not found
6. To encourage children to reflect on their experiences
7. To create a new role for the teacher, in which he or she becomes a resource rather than an authority.   Whitla, D. et al., 1970

The seven principal aims can be applied to any curriculum in any field of study. It is also pertinent to a vocational education where the development of a questioning attitude, using research methodology, reflecting on previous experiences, are all very important processes. But how are these processes to be inculcated into the curriculum?

Preparing for change – an experience of innovation

Experience has shown that before introducing a new curriculum, attention should be given to the preparation of those who are going to teach it. Many changes should and could have been brought about during the last two decades which could or would have paved the way for the implementation of Project

2000. For example, when I was the Director of Nurse Education at St. George's District School of Nursing in London, the following changes were implemented during the period between 1986–1990:

- In 1986, a deliberate policy of recruiting graduate nurse teachers was successfully introduced. By 1989, 75 per cent of the nurse teachers were graduates holding a range of academic and clinical specialisms.
- In 1987, one of the most enlightened English National Board for Nursing, Midwifery and Health Visiting (ENB) policies – 'the employment of non-nurse teachers in schools of nursing' was implemented. The curriculum of the school was enriched by the presence of two biological scientists, an occupational therapist, a lawyer, a tutor-librarian, a counsellor, a linguist, a family therapist and a behavioural therapist.
- The concept of subject teaching was introduced during 1989. This offered nurse teachers and non-nurse lecturers the opportunity to engage in their own academic and clinical specialisms.
- The strength of ward-based learning was recognised; a mentor system was introduced throughout the health authority using a quasi distance learning approach. The video tape made by the staff was an asset.
- In 1988, in collaboration with a college of higher education, a City and Guilds 730 Further Teachers and Adult Education Certificate was launched which received overwhelming interest from clinicians and supervisors.
- More importantly, deliberate curriculum changes were introduced which gave all the nursing students, at least during the first year of their training, a highly supervised status. For example: students undertaking the new mental health programme were in fact supernumerary; the post registration students spent 30 per cent of their study time in a college of higher education; conversion course students were offered the opportunity to study in a college of higher education. As a result of these changes, the new ethos of nurse education emerged.

Resourcing the curriculum

My experience has shown that before a new curriculum is introduced, great care should be given to the preparation of one of the most important human resources – those who will deliver it. The nurse teachers who took part in the Project 2000 National Foundation for Educational Research (NFER) research project appear to support this view (Jowett, et al., 1991). The following suggestions may help to implement a new curriculum in an organised way.

A series of curriculum workshops

There is considerable benefit in providing opportunities for teachers to understand the curriculum, to devise a learning and teaching strategy and to build up a repertoire of audio visual learning materials prior to introducing the new curriculum. The workshops also allow other groups of colleagues to participate in the implementation of a new course.

The course planning team should organise a series of curriculum workshops involving a range of staff, e.g. nurse teachers, supervisors, librarians, colleagues from higher education establishments. The workshops should be provided over a period of at least six months before the curriculum is implemented. The purpose of these workshops is to encourage staff to participate actively in curriculum development by allowing them to explore specific curriculum themes and to develop teaching materials and learning strategies for these themes.

Librarians should be allowed to take part in all these workshops as they will make a significant contribution to the future success of the course; not only will they help to bring the library stock up to date, assemble assessment materials and prepare appropriate teaching materials for seminars, project work etc., they will also contribute to some of the curriculum themes, e.g. study skills and research methodology.

The workshops will also allow teachers to iron-out any teething problems of the course. Some workshops might be used to bring people up to date with some of the ideas or concepts which have been introduced in the curriculum, e.g. inquiry based learning and continuous assessment.

Experience also shows that there is some value in bringing consultants in to help with these workshops. It costs money, but it works.

Educational supportive services

If student nurses of the new Project 2000 curriculum are to be given the opportunity to adopt inquiry-based learning, an adequate level of supportive services is assumed. Two types of educational supportive services in my view are essential to the needs of the student. These are:
– the library and information service;
– student counselling services.

The library and information service

There are ten criteria put forward in *Resourcing Project 2000 – the role of libraries* produced by the Nursing Information Subgroup of the Library Association and the Royal College of Nursing Library.
1. an environment conducive to learning with plenty of space, quiet rooms, private study carrels, and seminar rooms. Special attention should be paid to floor covering which should aim at reducing noise;
2. a range of books which should satisfy the intellectual rigour of the students, e.g. a student undertaking the mental health branch of nursing might require books on drama therapy, psychoanalysis;
3. a large number of journal titles;
4. facilities for inter-library loans – this raises the issue of whether the students should pay for these;
5. facilities for photocopying;
6. CD-Rom facilities;
7. AVA materials;
8. a satisfactory student/professional librarian ratio;
9. a satisfactory student/non professional library staff ratio;
10. a comprehensive and user friendly user education set.

The 10 criteria constitute the base line requirements of a comprehensive library and information service. A two part submission by the Library Association to the

All-Party Select Committee on Education, published in the May 1991 edition of the Library Association Record, recommended that each school library should have a minimum level of IT equipment consisting of:

- an online computer facility to access local data bases, education services;
- a CD-Rom workstation, to access NERIS, ECCTIS, electronic encyclopaedias, dictionaries and newspapers;
- interactive video;
- a desktop publishing workstation for the production of creative work;
- workstations where students can use software packages, word-processing, spreadsheets etc. in support of their curriculum work;
- commercial software packages;
- resource management systems capable of holding the records of the stock of learning materials.

Few, if any of the Colleges of Nursing and Midwifery have reached the standard recommended for schools in general education.

Student counselling services

From the students' viewpoint

Providing a comprehensive library and information service for student nurses undertaking the Project 2000 does not need a great deal of justification from the resources point of view as the benefits are immediately evident. However, a student counselling service might require some justification especially from the funding authorities' perspective.

There are several factors which might support the claim that there is a need to incorporate a student counselling service as part of the Project 2000 development. Firstly, it has been well documented that learning, taking assessments, examinations, are stress related activities. In Japan for example, the suicidal rate increases near examination periods. The feeling of not being able to cope or of lagging behind with assignments, are real concerns of students in any field of education. This ought to be recognised by funding authorities of Project 2000 courses.

There are other factors which can increase the stress level experienced by the student. As for any new initiative, new ideas are brought in and the implications of such ideas are not fully known especially from the experimental point of view – i.e. how it affects the recipient. For example, some of the Project 2000 curricula impose specific demands on students' time because of research based or inquiry based learning approaches. On the whole this type of learning consumes a great deal more time than listening to lectures, taking down notes at the time.

Because of the different learning/teaching strategies being adopted, the method of assessing students' competence will take on a different form. The students are required to produce assignments at specific times which can be stress-causing especially where bunching of assignments occurs. This can further engender feelings of worthlessness, not being able to cope, being under pressure. This may be compounded further by the fact that the Project 2000 is a new course. The teachers who teach on the course might also feel insecure in the way they approach the new subject areas which have been incorporated in the curriculum. This sets up a tension between teachers and students. Someone has to listen to their grumbles and dissatisfaction.

From the financial viewpoint

There are strong financial arguments to support the provision of a student counselling service in a Project 2000 college of nursing and midwifery. In the context of student retention, it is inevitable that a small percentage of any particular cohort of students will leave during the course of study for a variety of reasons. However, it is not cost effective to have a wastage of 30 per cent from any cohort of students. To produce a qualified nurse under the Project 2000 scheme, costs approximately £30,000 per student over a three year period. These costs include student bursary, teacher salary based on a student teacher ratio of 1:15 and the total running costs. A cohort of 80 students with a 30 per cent wastage rate will cost the country a great deal of money.

I undertook a project about four years ago primarily because of my concern to combat high wastage rate and high sickness and absence amongst student nurses in one of the schools of nursing. Employing a part-time student counsellor to combat a high wastage rate and high sickness and absence levels among student nurses had very positive results: the wastage rate went down from 25 per cent to 6 per cent within a couple of years. From the purely financial view point it is worth spending an extra £20,000 or so to employ a student counsellor in a college. In addition, student nurses will appreciate a friendly, unbiased ear.

Societal factors

There are several societal factors which might further support the case for a student counselling service. In the future, because of demographic changes students recruited for nursing will not be, by and large, school leavers; and nursing colleges are also in direct competition with higher education for the more able candidates. Colleges of nursing might have to adopt a different recruitment strategy than hitherto. From necessity as well as from sound educational and employment practice, a range of candidates with differing educational backgrounds might have to be recruited. Some of those recruited for the Project 2000 course might be less able than others, some might be older, and some might have been unemployed. These individuals will require additional support while undertaking a very demanding professional programme.

A dynamic environment

The term 'monotechnic' has been much to the fore during the last few years. Its negative connotations have worried some. There are a number of such establishments which are highly reputable within academic circles. Basically, there should be no problem in being monotechnic provided that the learning milieu is active and dynamic, that there is a variety of courses offered, and that there is a right mix of lecturing staff.

In principle, there are obvious benefits in being polytechnic as students are likely to be more exposed to different subject disciplines and opportunities for new experiences are greater. There are ways of eliminating some of the perceived educational problems of being a single discipline based educational establishment. About four years ago, two major changes were introduced at St. George's which transformed the single discipline based nursing education to multidisciplinary based nurse education. As said previously, the ENB non-Nurse lecturer policy was implemented. Financial resources were shifted from employing nurse teachers to employing other lecturers as the curriculum demanded. Eight new disciplines were introduced: biological sciences, occupational therapy, law, library information, counselling, physiotherapy, family therapy, behavioural therapy. As a result, the learning environment was enriched. The other significant change which we brought about was the introduction of subject teaching where the expertise of the sixty nurse teachers was classified based on their professional qualifications and clinical experiences. Through consultation with staff, a teaching matrix was organised so that teaching expertise was shared across all courses.

Although in principle a monotechnic nursing college can be transformed into a multidisciplinary organisation, a significant key factor might need to be taken into account, that is, the size of the college. A small college with about three to four hundred students would not be a viable proposition. The ability to introduce a new academic mix will also depend on the number of sites that the college has. A college with three or four sites separated by some distance would present a logistic problem, i.e. how to mobilise the staff in order to satisfy the demands of the curriculum, how to encourage staff and students to integrate.

Conclusion

Project 2000 offers a historic opportunity to remedy some of the educational problems experienced by both teachers and students. We are however entering into a period of instability where changes are brought in because of expediency to counteract financial difficulties. The concept of 'purchaser' and 'provider' offers a different dimension in the practice of nurse education. A medical school in London for example, in order to survive, is required to obtain 'training contracts' from a large number of health authorities. This is a worrying feature of the year 2000.

The other interesting question although it is not directly related to resource management, is nonetheless pertinent as it is concerned with the employability of our new product – the new type of practitioner, in the year 1992 and beyond. Should a European dimension be introduced into the new Project 2000 curriculum? If so, will colleges of nursing and midwifery be introducing European languages in the curriculum? These are also interesting resource questions. Will colleges of nursing be purchasing for example the expertise of linguists?

Expediency and short term gains may be attractive, but in the long term, students will be the losers, and the teachers will feel frustrated. Failure to achieve the curriculum aims intended will waste a great deal of time and effort.

References

Audit Commission. (1985). *Obtaining Better Value from Further Education: Report by the Audit Commission for Local Authorities in England and Wales*, London, HMSO
CNAA. (1989). *Towards an Educational Audit*, London, CNAA.

Balogh, R. and Beattie, A. (1988). *Performance Indicators in Nurse Education*, London, Institute of Education, University of London.

CVCP. (1986). *Performance Indicators in Universities: a First Statement by the Joint CVCP and UGC Working Group*, London, CVCP.

CVCP. (1987) *Performance Indicators in Universities: a Second Statement by the Joint CVCP and UGC Working Group*, London, CVCP.

Jowett, S., Walton, I. and Payne, S. (1991). *Interim paper No. 2, The NFER Project 2000 Research: an Introduction and Some Interim Issues*, Slough, NFER.

Library Association. (1991). *Library Association Record*, London, Library Association.

Whitla, D., Hanley, J.P., Moo, E.W. and Walter, A. (1970). *Man: A Course of Study: Education Strategies, Based on Research and Evaluation in the Educational Development Centre*. Washington DC, Curriculum Development Associates.

MacDonald, B. (1978). *The Experience of Innovation, Occasional Paper No. 6*, Centre for Applied Research in Education, Norwich, University of East Anglia.

Payne, S., Jowett, S. and Walton, I. (1991). I*nterim Paper No. 3, Nurse Teachers in Project 2000 – the Experience of Planning and Initial Implementation*, Slough, NFER.

Royal College of Nursing. (1992). RCN welcomes cash boost for Project 2000, Press release, London, RCN.

Sizer, J. (1979). Assessing institution performance – an overview, *International Journal of Institutional Management in Higher Education*, Vol. 3 (1): 49–75.

Sullivan, R.J. (1989). *Immanuel Kant's Moral Theory*, Cambridge, Cambridge University Press.

Stenhouse, L. (1975). *An Introduction to Curriculum Research and Development*, London, Heinemann.

Taylor, T. and Richard, C.M. (1985). *An Introduction to Curriculum Studies*, 2nd edition, Berkshire, NFER – Nelson Publishing Company Ltd.

10

Implementing Project 2000: the need for evaluation and review

Geoffrey Watts

Authors of novels or books which are eventually filmed frequently complain that the cinematic outcome bears little resemblance to the original story. There is a sense in which this is an apt analogy for the implementation of Project 2000.

The United Kingdom Central Council for Nursing, Midwifery and Health Visiting (UKCC), as original authors of the book, *Project 2000: a New Preparation for Practice* (UKCC, 1986) have watched the development of its 'story' pass through the hands of producers in the form of the National Boards to the Colleges and Institutions of Nurse Education who, since 1989, have been responsible for directing the implementation. To extend this analogy further, course planning teams have taken on the role of screen-writers, taking the concepts and ideas embodied within the original 'story' to produce a product with 'cinematic' impact. Insofar as Project 2000 will be on general release throughout the U.K. by the end of 1992, it is now appropriate to begin to question the extent to which Project 2000, 'the Movie', resembles the original story.

To raise questions concerning the relationship between a novel and a film, one is required to re-read the original story. Re-reading of the Project 2000 report reveals problems with a book-film analogy however and one must be mindful of the view of Stenhouse (1984), who, in reference to a culinary analogy he had used, suggested that: '… analogies should be abandoned before they cause indigestion'.

The reason for abandoning the book-film analogy for the implementation of Project 2000 is that the original report differed in a marked way from a novel. Novels usually contain structure, detail and often visual description and many examples could be cited from English Literature alone to illustrate this point. The opening chapter of *The Return of the Native* by Thomas Hardy, where he vividly describes the scene of Egdon Heath, is a cinematographers dream; but the Project 2000 report is not. *Project 2000: a New Preparation for Practice* did not set out to give structure, details or even visual description. Its stated purpose was only to guide and encourage movement in a general direction. It was essentially an interpretive document. Implicit within it was a recognition that although implementation throughout centres in the U.K. would be relatively similar, there would be local variation, determined by local resources and circumstances.

The fact that the UKCC did not set out to give fine detail, but only to guide and encourage a general direction was recognised by the English National Board for Nursing, Midwifery and Health Visiting (ENB, 1989) when it sought to establish the parameters within which interpretation should take place. The role of the ENB in 1989 was crucial to the implementation of Project 2000, and although mindful of Stenhouse's warning in relation to the use of analogy, the implementation of Project 2000 can be seen as also analogous to the great treks westwards to open up new lands in the United States, which occurred in the latter half of the last century. With this analogy, the role of the UKCC was to point in the general direction and exhort us to, 'Go west young man'. The ENB, however, sought to give some form of route-map and detail of necessary provisions that would be required en-route. The fact that it was a journey which hitherto had not been undertaken required the route-map and list of provisions to be treated with some caution.

To extend this particular analogy further, it must be recognised that although a very large number of institutions and colleges of nurse education have set off along the route since 1989, rather like wagon-trains heading out west, not even the first to set off have yet reached their destination. Given the uncertainty of the route there is also a danger that unless these 'wagon-trains', (especially those setting off first), constantly evaluate and review their course and progress, they are liable to lead each other into quicksand. This analogy serves to illustrate the need for early and constant evaluation and review of the course that implementation of Project 2000 has taken.

The need for early evaluation of Project 2000 is supported by the National Foundation for Educational Research (1991b) who have highlighted the difficulties that have been associated with implementation. These difficulties centre largely around the speed of implementation which the NFER considered detrimental to sound and careful planning. The NFER contrast how Project 2000 was implemented against how it may have been implemented by citing the view of Fullan who saw the implementation of educational change as an incremental process taking a minimum of 2–3 years. Fullan is cited as suggesting that:

'Effective implementation can only occur under conditions which allow individuals to react to the change, clarify their own meaning, form their own position and interact with other implementers in a process of re-socialisation which is at the heart of change'.

Fullan, 1982

The NFER Report concludes that it would appear few of these conditions were fulfilled with Project 2000 implementation. It is thus not surprising that in an earlier report (NFER, 1991a) the NFER describes the task of implementing Project 2000 in the first round districts as 'awesome'.

There exists a further and important reason why early and constant evaluation and review of Project 2000 should occur. At the risk of further indigestion this reason is again perhaps best illustrated through analogy.

If Project 2000 instead of being about innovation in nurse education, had been about innovation in aircraft construction, then what would have followed would have been a prolonged period of discussion, design and construction from blue-print. Following this would have been a lengthy period of rigorous flight-testing and modification before the award of a Certificate of Air-Worthiness. Although operating the new aircraft over a more prolonged period carrying passengers would have yielded further valuable evaluative information which would lead to modifications in design, the award of the Certificate of Air-Worthiness would at least have demonstrated that minimum design and safety requirements had been met from the outset.

Course design within the framework of Project 2000 has not, however, followed this model of approach. 'Certificates of Air-Worthiness', which, in the case of Project 2000 courses is professional and academic validation, have been awarded on production of a blue-print only, prior to construction and testing phases. Although this is a considerable act of faith by validating bodies, it presents a dilemma:

To what extent can modification and change be made to courses in the light of evaluation and review processes which reveal faults in design and construction, when validation has been awarded on the basis of the original blue-print? This dilemma raises questions relating to the amount of latitude course teams have in making modifications and the extent to which courses, once validated, become engraved on tablets of stone. It is important in the resolution of this dilemma for course management teams to be aware of the boundaries that professional and academic validation has set for them and to paraphrase a famous maxim: to have the grace to accept the things they cannot change; the courage to change the things they can; and the wit to know the difference.

Professional and academic validation is not a process of rigidly fixing a course in time and space. It may even be argued that validation is not a process of establishing boundaries or perimeters, but rather the formal marking out of an agreed starting point from which course management teams propose to progress, in which case it is then a question of judgement, of recognising what changes and modifications can, and indeed must, be made to avoid inertia; but at the same time avoiding change that is so far removed from the original ideas and concepts that it undermines the integrity of the original design.

To advocate early and constant evaluation and review requires a definition of that which is to be evaluated and reviewed. Essentially, the question is begged: Is it the process or the product? In its earlier report, the NFER (1991a), stated clearly that its research was concerned with the 'process' of implementation rather than its outcomes. This NFER Report suggested that: 'to investigate the impact of the Project 2000 reforms, a longer-term study of the career paths of those successfully completing the course would be required'.

It is apparent from this that evaluation and review should be directed not just at the educational courses that have been developed and implemented under the auspices of Project 2000, but also at the context within which these courses have been developed. This is to suggest that the organisation and logistics which surround course implementation must be subject to as much scrutiny at this early stage as the courses themselves.

It is because of this perceived differentiation between an educational course and the organisational and logistic infrastructure which supports a course, that the word 'curriculum' was omitted from the title of this chapter. A review of the educational literature tends to suggest that curriculum is usually defined in terms of planned educational experiences and intended student outcomes, the implication here being that curriculum innovation, (which requires evaluation and review) has occurred within a stable environment. The implementation of Project 2000, however, has been a process of major and rapid curriculum change within the context of changing organisational circumstances.

To have entitled this chapter 'the need for curriculum evaluation and review' would have been to suggest either that it is only course delivery that need be evaluated and reviewed; or that organisational and logistic issues relating to course design and delivery can be subsumed under the heading 'curriculum'. To suggest the latter would require the definition of the term 'curriculum' to be widened to something akin to the following: everything done in an educational institution and every way and circumstance in which it is done.

A further argument for widening the scope of evaluation and review of the implementation of Project 2000 is that conventional approaches to purely curriculum review do not normally seek to challenge underlying philosophies upon which curriculum innovation has been based. The Project 2000 report, however, contained and indeed it could be argued, was based upon a single key notion that was both radical and new at the time of publication: the notion of the 'knowledgeable doer'. This notion would appear to be universally accepted and is therefore uncontroversial as a basis for curriculum innovation. Nevertheless, notions regarding the process by which knowledgeable doers are developed require challenge. Since the publication of the Project 2000 Report in 1986, myriad assumptions have been formed regarding the meaning of the phase 'knowledgeable doer' and the means by which a state of 'knowledgeable doing' is achieved.

The concept of a knowledgeable doer presents as a philosophical problem and has to be seen in terms of a comparison between the intended outcomes of Project 2000 courses and conventional nurse training courses which Project 2000 was designed to replace. This comparison, however odious, is inevitable due to the fact that within the phrase 'knowledgeable doer' the emphasis is intended to be placed on the first word, thus giving a clear implication that the difference between conventional and Project 2000 courses is intended to be within the cognitive domain.

This raises the issue as to whether differences in the psycho-motor (doing) domain are expected to manifest as a result of Project 2000. Indeed the whole notion of the inter-relationship of theory ·and practice in nursing is raised by this debate. Is knowledge about nursing and the doing of nursing inextricably linked, or are they discrete elements which are capable of individual development?

This question of the nature of nursing or nursing-related knowledge and nursing practice, and the extent to which comparison can be made between the outcomes of conventional and Project 2000 courses may be illustrated albeit simply, by the following figures:

Figure 1 is intended to represent skill acquisition learning curves for conventional students (Curve (a)) and Project 2000 student (Curve (b)).

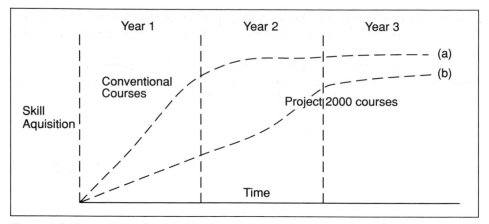

Figure 1 Skill acquisition learning curves

Curve (a) suggests that due to service commitment in conventional courses and hence a significantly greater proportion of time spent in a limited number of mostly institutional placement settings, conventional students had a more rapid skills learning curve than is expected from their Project 2000 counterparts.

Curve (b) suggests that Project 2000 students' learning curve for skill acquisition will be slower until much further into the course, but will eventually climb steeply to match the height of conventional students at the end of the course.

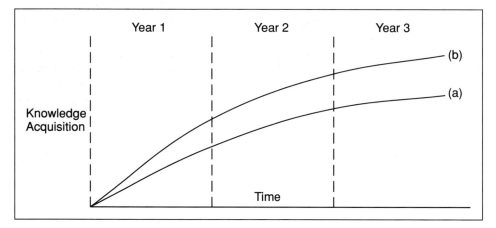

Figure 2 Knowledge acquisition learning curves

Figure 2 is intended to represent knowledge acquisition learning curves for conventional students (curve (a)) and Project 2000 students (curve (b)).

Although both curves suggest a linear development of knowledge during a three year period, the figure suggests that the knowledge acquisition learning curve for Project 2000 students is steeper and will rise higher than that of conventional students. It must be emphasised that the difference in these learning curves is seen as attributable to Project 2000 students having greater time and access to sources of knowledge, as well as greater depth of knowledge, rather than being attributable to any difference in the abilities of conventional and Project 2000 students.

If these basic suppositions which are illustrated in Figures 1 and 2 are accepted, then the notion of knowledgeable doing as an outcome of Project 2000 presents a dilemma illustrated in Figures 3 and 4.

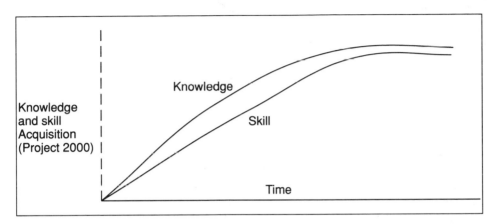

Figure 3 Development of knowledge and skill acquisition (Project 2000)

Figures 3 and 4 are essentially illustrative presentations of two differing hypotheses regarding the relationship of the development of knowledge and skill acquisition for Project 2000 students.

Figure 3 represents the following hypothesis: that there is a direct correlation between knowledge and skill acquisition. As the knowledge base develops, it enhances the skill acquisition. Further; that as skill acquisition develops, it informs and develops the knowledge base so that knowledge and skill acquisition are essentially symbiotic; developing and feeding off each other.

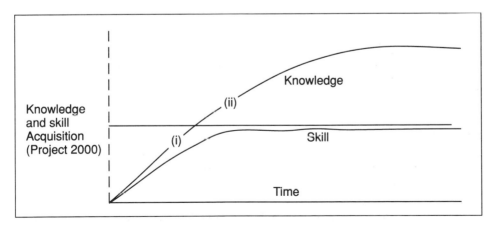

Figure 4 Development of knowledge and skill acquisition (Project 2000)

171

Figure 4 represents a second hypothesis which states that the hypothesis illustrated in Figure 3 only holds true to a certain point on the knowledge/skill acquisition learning curves but that eventually a point is reached, illustrated by the horizontal plane on the figure, when further knowledge acquisition does not affect the skill acquisition learning curve.

Knowledge gained on the learning curve above the horizontal plane is therefore of a different type to that on the learning curve below the horizontal plane. Knowledge below the horizontal plane is labelled type (i) knowledge, and knowledge above the horizontal plane is labelled type (ii) knowledge. This second hypothesis suggests that whereas type (i) knowledge conforms to the first hypothesis in that it is directly correlated to the skill acquisition learning curve and vice-versa, type (ii) knowledge, rather than enhancing skill acquisition, serves other purposes. These other purposes may be seen as conferring confidence on the learner (or even enhancing esteem or status). It may enable the learner to reflect on practice and be more analytical and critical in relation to practice but does not necessarily enhance practice performance *per se*.

It may be argued that this concept of knowledgeable doing is the single most important aspect of the implementation of Project 2000 that course teams must come to terms with. Unless it is addressed at an early stage of implementation through processes of evaluation and review, a danger exists that future course curriculum planning will tend to concentrate on developing in the academic domain only. As nurse education continues to collaborate and even merge with higher education, the ever increasing requirement for the demonstration of academic rigour in courses of nurse education may obscure the need to clearly define the expected nature and level of clinical practice.

If the level of practice expected of a Project 2000 graduand is indeed perceived as at least comparable with those completing conventional courses, then the question which will inevitably be asked is what is this increased knowledge base ultimately for? Evaluation and review of courses are the processes by which course teams must begin to resolve the issue of how this increased knowledge base provided by Project 2000 course will manifest in clinical practice.

The main tenet of this chapter has been to advocate early and continual evaluation and review of the implementation of Project 2000. It is appropriate, however, to address certain broad issues, which relate specifically to course evaluation. The Council for National Academic Awards (CNAA), who have been the joint validation body with the English National Board for a considerable number of Project 2000 courses, see course evaluation as a process of critical appraisal. The CNAA (1987) suggests a number of dimensions to course evaluation, which, when applied to Project 2000 courses, may be summed up into three broad issues which, it may be suggested, would benefit from early critical appraisal: the theoretical component of courses, the practical component of courses and teaching activity within Project 2000.

The theoretical component of courses

Reference was made earlier to the fact that the UKCC in its original report, sought only to give broad direction in relation to the implementation of Project 2000, more specific guidance in relation to course structure and context being

172

provided by the National Boards (cf. ENB 1989). Within the guidelines and criteria for course development established by the National Boards the requirement that courses established under the auspices of Project 2000 should comprise 50% of full-time academic study was, arguably, the most significant challenge faced by course planning teams. The National Boards requirement that Project 2000 courses should be contained within a three year period, resulted in courses being planned in which the amount of time available for academic teaching and study increased in relation to conventional courses by a factor of three. It was undoubtedly a consolation to planning teams that the National Boards endeavoured to give some detailed guidance in relation to what should constitute the content, at least in outline, of the academic component. The manner in which this outline content or syllabus was utilised by course planning teams was determined, largely, by the particular course structure and curriculum philosophy adopted by course teams.

Despite differing curricular approaches which were available to course teams, from relatively straightforward linear models to more complex modular and/or integrated approaches, all course planning teams were faced with confronting two challenges viz: the need to provide 'vertical cohesiveness' and 'academic progression' within their particular course plan.

Vertical cohesiveness relates to the need to consider how individual subjects or topics should be taught on a day to day basis. A course structure that allowed for the teaching of discrete units of differing social and physical sciences relevant to nursing allowed planning teams to make specific choices within units of study in terms of content and sequencing. A potential danger however, does exist with this approach, in that planning within these units of study was liable to occur without any cross-reference to planning and decision taking within other units, this lack of relationship or coherence vertically across the units being liable to inculcate in student minds, the view that within the academic component, the whole of the course was simply the sum of the parts, with little requirement to integrate or even relate subject matter. A course structure which allows the development of discrete units of academic study with little, if any, inter-relationship renders the concept of theory-practice integration problematic. Although teaching staff delivering those units may make bold attempts to relate their particular subject matter to clinical nursing practice, without some form of cross-discipline co-ordination the outcome is liable to be confusion in the minds of the students. Cross-discipline co-ordination to relate theory to practice must, of necessity, be led by the discipline of nursing studies which directs the application of the other disciplines towards practice. In this sense, the discrete units of study can be envisaged as being arranged like ducks in flight; with nursing studies at the point of the chevron, leading and determining direction.

The second challenge that faces planning teams, that of ensuring academic progression across the course, relates less to providing the students with access to more complex information as the course progresses, but more to what students should be able to achieve intellectually as they progress. This intellectual expectation must of course be related to the academic level to which the course is written; be it certificate, diploma or degree.

Since the first Project 2000 courses were implemented in late 1980s/1990 in

England, academic validation, with one or two notable exceptions has been awarded at Higher Education Diploma level. Within a year of implementation of the first Project 2000 courses the CNAA were concerned to give guidance as to what should be seen as diploma-worthy. In considering the level of courses, the CNAA were to comment that:

> 'Many nurses seem to be seeking some precise definition of diploma level and do not find it helpful to be told this is in advance of certificate level but not yet degree level.'   CNAA, 1991

In seeking to clarify the notion of diploma level, the CNAA guidance notes expressed the view that at diploma level, students should be able to use knowledge accurately and apply it appropriately to the practice of nursing, they should have the beginnings of informed critical comment and a level of analytical thinking which enables them to progress into degree level work.

This guidance was at least an attempt to mark out the finishing point of Project 2000 courses, on the basis of which course teams needed to work backwards to establish the stages through which students could be expected to pass *en-route* to this end goal. In determining this route of progress for students, it was also necessary to determine the formative and summative theoretical assessment strategies through which this academic progression could be both measured and monitored. Assessment strategies, however, can only measure academic progress and contribute little if anything to an understanding of the issues of course structure, content or disciplinary cohesiveness. Course teams are obliged to develop evaluation and review strategies to address these issues at an early stage in order that they progress with confidence with course delivery as implementation of Project 2000 unfolds.

The practical component of courses

The concept of supernumerary status embodied within Project 2000 meant that it was possible for course planning teams to consider the provision of practice experience in an imaginative and innovative way, which hitherto had been hindered by the demands of service commitment. Indeed, it may be argued that without a high degree of flair and imagination, course teams would not have been able to fulfil the complex requirements the National Boards outlined in their guidance documentation. To provide across a common foundation programme alone, a wide variety of institutional, non-institutional NHS and private sector experience, as well as a range of specialist, branch-focused, experience for cohorts of up to and beyond 100 students has required knowledge, organisational skill and tenacity of purpose of an exceptionally high level. Given the speed of implementation of Project 2000 since late 1989, one must marvel, not that colleges of nursing have achieved this feat well in all instances, but that they have managed to achieve it at all.

Whilst achievement must be recognised and acknowledged, there is a need to guard against complacency. To provide a wide and varied quantity of placement activity for students is not necessarily to provide a high quality of experience; although it must be recognised that the two are not mutually exclusive. It is important that through the processes of evaluation and review, questions are asked regarding the extent to which placement activity is achieving its aim. Providing students with supernumerary clinical experience is about much more than giving well-earned breaks from college. It is about providing an experience which enables professional growth and development of competent, independent practitioners. It is about making the theoretical component come alive and meaningful so that students may relate their studies in a way which informs their practice. Unless course teams develop sound methods of preparing students for practice experiences, these ideals in relation to practice will become no more than glib rhetoric. As Project 2000 frees course planners from the bonds of service commitment, it is no longer necessary for practice experience to be presented as periods of prolonged allocation to a very limited number of placement areas. Project 2000 has allowed course teams to consider carefully the nature of the experience available in each potential placement area, the range of learning outcomes achievable and the actual amount of time which it is likely a student would require to achieve those outcomes. It is inevitable that this has resulted in many instances with patterns of placement experience which are radically different from the 'modular' pattern of placement, so much a feature of traditional courses.

Whatever the advantages of these placement patterns that are emerging as a result of Project 2000, they do present with some significant concerns. One over-riding concern is that as time available for practice experience with Project 2000 has reduced considerably in comparison with conventional courses, what criteria should be used in choosing clinical placement areas so that students are provided with a qualitative experience? Applied to this must be a concern in relation to ensuring a progression in clinical nursing skill development. It is essential that students who undergo a larger number of relatively shorter periods of placement are able to transfer learning as well as apply and adapt that learning to new situations. It must not be assumed that transfer of learning will occur naturally. Unless students are encouraged to see the totality of the practice experience and are assisted to make the links between those experiences, there exists the danger that students will perceive this pattern of practice experience as a series of short, fragmented and totally unrelated episodes.

The need for sound and effective preparation in relation to the practice component of Project 2000 courses is no less true in the case of clinical staff charged with the responsibility of supervising, mentoring and assessing students. Speed of implementation has again meant that opportunities for dialogue, negotiation and discussion have been severely limited. This must also be coupled with the fact that implementation of Project 2000 has coincided with enormous change within service areas, who have traditionally supported nurse training courses. The advent of NHS Trusts, managerial re-organisations, skill-mix changes and changes related to the allocation of finance and other resources have understandably placed new courses developed within the framework of Project 2000 rather low on the list of health service priorities. At the same time however, awareness of these new courses, but lack of knowledge or understanding about their nature, is likely to have engendered more apprehension than anticipation in the minds of service staff. It should not be assumed that trained staff will adjust to the demands of this new body of students without knowing what their new learning needs are and how they differ from those with which they have traditionally been involved.

The manner in which students of nursing are taught, supervised and assessed during clinical practice has been steeped with assumption for many years. Since the mid 1970s many studies have emerged which sought to examine clinical learning environments. Studies by Orton (1981), Fretwell (1980) and Ogier (1981) have examined learning climates, how they are orientated towards students and how senior nursing staff can influence and play a role in establishing learning climates. In a later study, however, Watts (1988) has suggested that although a positive student-orientated climate is conducive for students in clinical areas, it should not be assumed that such climates increase the extent to which students are supervised or taught.

It is possible that such climates serve only to increase students confidence in soliciting help, guidance or information when practising with only a form of 'distant-supervision' being provided. The use of a system of distance-supervision, which requires students to solicit support when required ignores the fact that it requires a student to be aware of his/her lack of knowledge or skill. A student who is unsure of his/her practice will quickly solicit guidance given that there exists a conducive learning climate in the clinical area. But even the most student-orientated clinical climate is unhelpful to a student who does not know, but does not know he/she does not know.

If supervision of students has traditionally been in the form of 'distant-supervision' because of the expediency of work-loads and students being part of the work-force (with the consequence that assessment of skills development has been largely by inference) then this fact must be recognised and addressed. Project 2000 students, at least during early practice experiences, are highly unlikely to have the necessary confidence and skill required to cope with this form of clinical supervision. Current changes in skill-mix in NHS establishments are unlikely to enhance the capacity of trained staff to closely support and monitor Project 2000 students during their supernumerary periods of practice. It is only through a prolonged process of dialogue with trained staff that methods of supervision, teaching and assessment of students can be evaluated and reviewed to ensure that with the advent of Project 2000, methods of supervision and support for students are refined and developed to meet their particular needs.

Teaching activity within Project 2000

Project 2000 is without doubt the biggest change to affect nursing in seventy years, and for those involved in implementing its educational changes, the amount of change has been of a magnitude barely imaginable even as late as 1988. What has been achieved to date must be seen as a tribute to the commitment of those involved in this venture. The nature of the new courses are such that teaching staff have been required to adapt and adjust to new teaching styles and methods of course delivery, in an extremely short time period.

But Project 2000 has required teaching staff to cope with much more than this. From a tradition of being generecists, nurse teachers have rapidly had to adopt the role of subject specialists as the new course curricula have been developed. They have also had to develop more appropriate teacher-student relationships as they become confronted with a student body with an entirely different self-perception than that of traditional students.

The speed of implementation has again meant that nurse teachers have been obliged to cope with these changes with minimal, if any, staff development opportunities. Many staff have developed via totally experiential learning, managing and coping with the changes on a daily basis. It is because of this fact, that it would be wrong to ignore the human cost; and to assume that this change is not problematic.

Teacher activity within Project 2000 must be as amenable to evaluation and review as any other aspect addressed in this chapter. The evaluation and review of teaching activity must, however, be a positive and constructive process. It must seek to help support and develop teaching staff to their full potential. Educational literature abounds with advice regarding the differing approaches which may be adopted to the evaluation of teacher activity. Although the merits of student evaluation and self-evaluation are recognised as important contributors to the process, the newness of Project 2000 and the anxieties and apprehensions which are associated with its implementation would suggest that the most valuable and constructive method is that of peer evaluation.

Project 2000 has seen a widespread increase in team teaching methods as a response to increased cohort sizes, which lends itself to methods of peer evaluation. Evaluation by peers tends to be more honest, constructive and mutually supportive. It is also frequently reported to be far less destructive than evaluation by students. Peer evaluation also has the very positive benefit of avoiding the problems associated with subjectivity in self-evaluation. Peer evaluation is also self-regulative. It empowers teachers to evaluate and review their contribution; as such, it tends not to be seen as an imposition by those in authority.

Peer evaluation is likely to make a significant contribution to staff development as colleges undertake the transition from conventional to Project 2000 courses. It is important that senior college staff have the courage and confidence to allow those delivering the course to monitor, evaluate and review their own activity.

Conclusion

In summary, this chapter has attempted to address the issues of evaluation and review without attempting to be prescriptive about methods adopted. Methods can only be developed that are appropriate to local needs and circumstances.

Evaluation and review is ultimately about asking the right questions in the right way, and as such, is akin to the research process. The process of research is, in fact, anticipated by processes of evaluation and review, and Project 2000 affords nursing enormous opportunity to further develop its research base, in practice, as well as education.

The direction and destination of Project 2000 must be constantly questioned; the price for not doing so will be nurse education wandering aimlessly in the wilderness, an activity few survive for long.

References

Council for National Academic Awards. (1987). *Handbook*, London, CNAA.

Council for National Academic Awards. (1991). *Draft Notes for Guidance Regarding the Design and Validation of Project 2000 Dip. H.E. Nursing Courses*, London, CNAA.

ENB. (1991). *Circular 74, Comments of the English National Board on Draft Notes for Guidance Regarding the Design and Validation of Project 2000 Dip. H.E. Nursing Courses*, London, ENB.

ENB. (1989). *Project 2000: A New Preparation for Practice: Guidelines and Criteria for Course Development and the Formation of Collaborative Links between Approved Training Institutions within the National Health Service and Centres of Higher Education,* London, ENB.

Fretwell J. (1980). An enquiry into the ward learning environment, *Nursing Times*, Vol. 76 No. 16, 69–73.

Fullan M. (1982). *The Meaning of Educational Change*, New York, Teachers College Press.

NFER. (1991a). *The NFER Project 2000 Research, an Introduction and some Interim Issues, National Evaluation of Demonstration Schemes in Pre-registration Nurse Education, Interim Paper 2,* Slough, NFER.

NFER. (1991b). *Nurse Teachers in Project 2000, the Experience of Planning and Initial Implementation, National Evaluation of Demonstration Schemes in Pre-registration Nurse Education, Interim Paper 3,* Slough, NFER.

Ogier, M. (1981). Ward Sisters and their influence upon nurse learners, *Nursing Times*, Vol. 77 No. 11, 41–43.

Orton, H. (1981). Ward learning climate and student nurse response, *Nursing Times*, Vol. 77 No. 17, 65–68.

Stenhouse, L. (1984). *An Introduction to Curriculum Research and Development,* London, Heinemann.

UKCC. (1986). *Project 2000: A new preparation for practice,* London, UKCC.

Watts, G.E. (1988). Learning nursing; the development of theory relating to student nurses practical learning experiences, Unpublished M.Ed. Dissertation, Crewe & Alsager College of Higher Education.

11

Beyond be dragons

Patricia Scott

Remember the old maps labelled 'here be dragons'? I thought I did too, and once tried to obtain a print of one of those old maps to use in a lecture. I will not bore you with the details of the ensuing research, but I was seriously disappointed to discover, as far as any of the multiple informants consulted could tell, such maps never existed: the legend is apocryphal. Never mind; nurses are adaptable and the concept can still serve as an illustration.

The idea, of course, was that beyond the boundaries of the explored world, dragons lay in wait, and these unknown places were to be avoided. Ancient mariners navigated their ships, more or less safely, from one known point to another, until 500 years ago, when Columbus came along and changed all that. Contrary to what a lot of people were sure they knew, Columbus believed he could sail *west* to reach the *eastern* side of India. The records do not tell us what he thought about dragons, but for the sake of the illustration, let us indulge a little fantasy and assume he 'knew' they were out there, but with the prospect of cheaper exotic spices, he was prepared to take the risk. Columbus was prepared to adventure. He did not accept there were 'places to be avoided'.

The dictionary defines adventure, in part, as 'risk, danger, daring enterprise, hazardous activity'. Columbus was daring. This chapter, *Beyond be dragons*, is a personal view of nursing from a perspective of intellectual adventure. Nursing in the year 2000 and beyond is uncharted, unmapped territory. Nursing is a developing profession; the boundaries extend daily. None of us are sure in 1992 exactly where the boundaries are, or exactly what is encompassed in the domain of nursing. Columbus found adventure in exploring uncharted areas. I suggest that we as nurses, in exploring and mapping the domain of nursing, not only can but should engage in intellectual activities that may be as risky, as dangerous, as daring, as hazardous and as much *fun* as any other kind of exploration and discovery. Beyond the known, mapped, safe territory we know as nursing – beyond be dragons. The dragons, of course, are as apocryphal as the rest of the story, symbolic of the fear of the unknown.

> The world of the year 2000 will be far more different from the world of 1980 than the world of 1980 was from 1780 ... and the future beyond will be almost unimaginably different from the twentieth century.　　　Platt, 1980

One author (Christman, 1976) sees the role *components* that cut across all professions as service, education, consultation and research. As far as nursing is concerned, most of us would add management to the list. Although I believe consultation is a separate role in its own right, for the purposes of this paper, I include consultation as a component in all nursing roles. In my view these four major components provide a very useful way for looking at what we do. I am a nurse. My primary identity is in the 'nurse' role. I am also an academic in the sense that what I do about nursing these days takes place for the most part within an academic environment, but I do not care much for the dictionary definition of an academic: 'Scholarly (and by implication) abstract; unpractical; cold; merely logical.' If those of us in the profession (I use the term loosely) were not committed to nursing, what would we be scholarly and abstract about? My academic identity supports my professional identity. I am puzzled by the occasional remark that someone 'used to be a nurse'. Nursing is not just something I do – a nurse is what I am. I am committed to the development of nursing as an academic, scientific discipline; inherent in this commitment is a passion for excellence in the profession. Passion may sound out of place in such a context, but for me it is passion which enables risk-taking, which transforms what is sometimes ordinary, everyday plodding into adventures. The excitement and the adventure are at the outer edges, on the frontiers of what is known.

As we move towards the year 2000, let us examine the frontiers which cover the four role components, within a framework derived from *A Strategy for Nursing, Midwifery and Health Visiting in Northern Ireland* (DHSS, 1991).

Nursing practice

The first Strategy statement is on practice and begins:

> 'The nursing profession is an integral part of a multi-disciplinary team working towards a common patient or client-centred goal.' DHSS, 1991

The turf dragons

We meet our first dragons, the *Fighting Over Our Turf Dragons*. What turf is ours? Which activities are rightfully on nursings' turf and which belong more properly to other members of the multi-disciplinary team? What is nursing's domain? Since 1978 the International Council of Nursing has been trying to devise a definition of nursing acceptable to all member countries, with a singular lack of success. An unmapped territory? I suggest it is. What makes nursing *nursing* and not something else? After all, there would be no 'turf battles' if we had clear title to our territory. If we examine what nurses are *seen* to do we can understand why I ask the question, and why these particular dragons introduce this section. Patients and physicians, according to Kramer (1974) tend to describe nurses primarily in terms of manual activities. Bosk (1980) and Wolf (1988) identifying what are described as the 'major occupational rituals' of nursing, single out medication administration, medical asepsis procedures and the 'hands on' physical care involved in providing whatever is required for personal hygiene, from bathing to toileting. If we think about them, none of these manual activities are unique or peculiar to nursing. Many scientists use 'sterile' techniques to avoid contamination, as do many cooks in home canning and preserving. The administration of medications by nurses is held to be almost sacred; yet people have been medicating themselves for centuries. I could go on, but you get the general idea. A major task for nursing is to define what is uniquely *nursing* in such a way that the boundaries are clear to ourselves, our patients and our colleagues.

The activity dragons

These dragons, *Superdragon* and *Do Everything Dragon*, are very closely related to the *Turf Dragons*; it might be useful to consider activities and turf together. I believe it is our identification of our *activities* (hands on 'doing'; meeting all our patients' needs) with our *domain* which has led to much confusion among ourselves regarding our boundaries.

How central are activities in the realm of professional nursing? For years nurses have been saying it is the 'art, science and spirit' (Harmer and Henderson, 1939; Emmerson and Taylor, 1950; Brunner, et al., 1974) with which nurses perform activities which make the difference; laudable, perhaps, but it hardly answers the question.

More recent authors (Fox, et al., 1990; Holzemer, 1991) talk of the science of caring. But caring is not unique to nursing. If we believe Rogers (1970), the purpose of professional education is to provide the knowledge and tools whereby individuals may become artists in their chosen field.

> Patient care cannot be improved by nurses who have expert psychomotor skills but lack a background in science any more than it can be improved by persons who have complete theoretical knowledge but lack the expert psychomotor skills necessary to transform that knowledge into quality nursing care.   Christman, 1976

The 'art' of nursing has an intellectual aspect: discerning and planning for what can and should be done, plus the practical aspect of actually doing it. The practical aspects of nursing can often be delegated; the intellectual aspects cannot. This, I believe, brings us to perhaps the major unexplored frontier, some might say a precipice.

The domain of nursing is defined, I believe, by the *phenomena* of concern to nurses: human responses to actual or potential health problems (O'Toole and Loomis, 1989). Human responses encompass biological (physiological, if you prefer), cognitive, affective and motor behaviours. These behaviours may or may not be due to identifiable stimulation, but they can be observed.

In my view, caring and doing, though of absolutely crucial importance, do not make nursing a science. The caring and doing can begin to become scientific activities when guided by clinical judgements – the nurses' own clinical judgements. Observations on the cognitive and affective behaviours as well as on the more traditional physiological and motor behaviours are organised into categories.

No one seems to have any problem with identifying these observations as 'assessments'. These assessments can be grouped and used by clinicians to formulate nursing diagnoses, which is simply the name for the aggregate or pattern of human responses. Nursing diagnoses are important because they provide direction, the rationale, for nursing interventions. The diagnosis is the judgment the nurse makes on the basis of the evidence.

Many nurses object strenuously to the use of the term 'diagnosis'. Diagnosing is often thought to be treading on somebody else's turf. But why? Diagnosis is not wholly owned by any group or profession. The local mechanic uses a machine to diagnose electronically what is wrong with my car; the plumber diagnoses what is wrong with the leaky pipe; beauty consultants diagnose what is wrong with complexions; why should nurses not diagnose in their domain? I would welcome another word for the process that would keep everybody happy, but is it *the word* or *the process* that is really objectionable? I fail to see how nurses can proceed to intelligent interventions (our jargon for action) without going through the process, and it is this process of clinical decision making which distinguishes us from non-nurses who carry out the same activities. The clinical decision-making cannot be delegated; only nurses can make judgments about their own domain. Exploring these domains more fully seems to me one of the most exciting and adventurous prospects in nursing today.

Nursing education

We move on to the Strategy statement on education, and see what dragons await. The statement declares that:

> Education must be responsive and relevant to the needs of patients, clients, practitioners and employers. Quality of care is directly linked to quality of education. It is essential that care is delivered by a confident, flexible and competent practitioner whose practice is, where possible, research based. All registered practitioners must take every reasonable opportunity to improve their education and practice with a personal commitment to lifelong education.
>
> DHSS, 1991

The traditional dragon

Immediately we encounter the much revered *Tradition Dragon*, enthroned on the altar of tradition, surrounded by an entire tribe of *We've Always Done it This Way Dragons.*

As Bevis pointed out in 1982, the great dilemma of nursing educators is that no one knows what information will survive in the rapid validation and generation process occurring in the physical, biological and social sciences today. Another difficult problem for the information-oriented curriculum is that for many years learning psychologists have demonstrated definitively that less than 25 percent of current material 'learned' is available for recall in two years, unless it is used and reinforced regularly or organised around meaningful life processes.

The knowledge nursing students should be encouraged to acquire is not only that 'useful for the moment' but a firm base from which they can explore new roads, new horizons, new territories, and continue to develop nursing knowledge which is relevant for the future. Building a theoretical knowledge base in nursing demands:

'...creative minds, intellectual superiority, and broad knowledge. Logic and reasoning are essential ingredients. Skill in simple problem solving and the development of mechanical devices are not to be confused with the complexity of creative thinking that must provide the concepts integral to professional growth. Nursing research is oriented to seeking further truths and understandings about life process.... It will not arise out of mere observation, but must evolve from intellectual processes   Rogers, 1970

Education must demonstrate to students how to use resources to gain new knowledge and how to implement research studies relevant to their practice so the findings can be validated and improved, knowledge gained and shared. We must create a climate conducive to intellectual adventure. Proust said 'The real voyage of discovery consists not in seeking new lands, but in seeing with new eyes.' We have to get around the dragons of tradition in order to do that. If I may be permitted to skip around the strategy document a bit, let us return to the Practice Strategy, and we read under Statement 4:

'Nurses must be adaptable and innovative in their approach to nursing care, particularly in relation to changing needs and advances in treatment. These advances may raise ethical, moral and environmental issues for nursing.'
                                                                                          DHSS, 1991

Consider these key points with me: knowledgeable, receptive, thinking, rational, critical, ethical and moral. According to Vito, (1983) 'many nursing educators and curriculum theory developers have accepted the responsibility for preparing nurses for ethical, moral and humanistic practice.' John Dewey (1909) suggests education should consist of supplying the conditions which will enable the psychological functions of the student to mature. Plato advocated exposing children to conflicts to develop character; he postulated that blind, habitual morality leaves individuals unable to cope with novel situations. (Livingstone, 1958). The cognitive developmental approach is directed toward developing abilities in problem solving and decision making. 'Moral development is not an increasing knowledge of cultural values but the transformations that occur in the individual's structure of thought' (Vito, 1983, p. 109). Florence Nightingale did wonderful things in originating the development of nursing as a profession, but the legacy left to nursing education produced nurses who did as they were told, adding a professionally submissive role to the traditionally submissive female role. 'Professional submissiveness is a contradiction in terms' (Cohen, 1981). Group and Roberts (1974) suggested that we have to exorcise the ghost of the Crimea, that nursing still maintains an authoritarian and militaristic structure, and that this interferes with the development of autonomy and critical thinking.

   Exorcising the ghost of the Crimea means we have to enable students to reach a high level of moral thinking. Scholars have written on moral development in higher education over the last three decades, but particularly in the 1970s (Kohlberg, 1976, 1978; Trow, 1976; Barnett, 1978; Brown and Carron, 1978; Blinder, 1977) among others. Studies abound which suggest that we need not, in higher education, concern ourselves too much with the preconventional level I. Most entering students are in level II, the conventional level, where moral

183

value resides in performing good or right roles, in maintaining the conventional order and the expectancies of others – exactly where Florence wanted them to be. In level III, the postconventional level, moral value resides in conformity by the self to shared standards, rights or duties and the orientation is to conscience as the directing agent.

Blatt's work (supervised by Kohler, 1978) is of particular interest to nurse educators: his findings indicate that transition to the next higher stage of moral development is most likely to happen when young people are challenged with moral dilemmas for which their stage of thinking provides no easy solutions, when they are presented with processes at the next higher stage and when they are able to work through progressive elaboration of the cognitive structures by experience. Nursing education today is really 'into' experiential learning; this frontier of moral development as an aid to learning critical thinking should, I believe, have a high priority for further exploration.

Nursing research

So on to the next frontier; Research. The Strategy is admirably concise: 'Research underpins all nursing development.' Statement 1 declares:

'Research should be encouraged as a continuing activity in enhancing nursing practice, education and management and in shaping its future.'   DHSS, 1991

The knowledge dragon

The *Research-based Knowledge Dragon* is one of the most pervasive. In keeping with the frontier approach, we will pass over the usual 'known' research and explore round the edges of emerging concepts.

Nursing knowledge is simultaneously the laws and the relationships existing between the elements that describe the phenomena of concern in nursing (factual knowledge) and the laws or rules that the nurse uses to combine the facts to make clinical nursing decisions. An example of factual knowledge is knowledge established by research. An example of the laws is the expert's 'rules of thumb' for practice (Graves and Corcoran, 1989).

Not many nursing phenomena can be measured in precise terms. In the first place, many of the phenomena are 'fuzzy' – the property of fuzziness of an entity, according to Zadek, (1978) is the result of the fact that the transition from membership to nonmembership in the class is not abrupt, but gradual. For example, 'strong' is a concept of interest to nurses checking neurological signs. One infant may have a strong grip, another weak; how does one compare infant grips with those of an adult male bricklayer? What about 'tall'? Height can be measured in inches but how tall is tall? Is a six-foot woman tall? or just 'tall for a woman'? The nurse must not only have solid ideas of the measures 'tall' and 'strong' but must know something about females and males, about babies and adults. This adds a second property, context dependence. In nursing research, much richness and meaning lie in fuzziness and context. There is perhaps a greater scope for qualitative research on the frontiers of nursing knowledge when one is still defining the variables. Qualitative does not mean lacking in rigour. To categorise observations reliably, we must have a requirement for rigour in operational definitions of observations. The observation 'has a good appetite' tells us nothing about nutritional status: one can have a good appetite and eat nothing. To date, the study of clinical inference has been poorly supported in nursing. We know very little about what or how data and information are used by clinicians in measuring complex and fuzzy phenomena (Corcoran, 1986).

Research-based knowledge is all about developing expertise in practice. Expertise in nursing requires the development of a repertoire of clinical judgements. This is extremely difficult to do. Is bleeding moderate or severe? Besides depending on the *context* (a tablespoon from a finger is severe, but negligible in abdominal surgery) it depends on the *experience* of the nurse within the particular context. Benner's (1984) work suggests expert clinical judgement develops through prolonged (10 years plus) experience in similar patient populations; despite the research base one still encounters curricula which expect expertise to be developed through courses. Theoretical content can at best provide the underpinnings; there is no substitute for experience.

As we move into the next century, information technology systems (programmes plus computers) will be used increasingly to manage and process information for nursing research. Already nursing researchers acknowledge four *ways of knowing* as being crucial to nursing practice: empirical, ethical, personal and aesthetic (Carper, 1978). Kramer and Chinn (1988) have elaborated on Carper's patterns of knowing. Each knowledge pattern is defined by a conceptual description and also by what can be considered 'permissible processing operations', parameters, conditions and methods for generating, verifying and transmitting each pattern of knowing. We can use information technology when we can model our thinking and decision making processes more accurately. One can then assume 'knowledge typing' – and study of this knowledge typing in nursing is expected to influence significantly the design of expert decision support systems. The use of models in information technology may require rearrangement of the thinking in some nursing circles on 'models and theories', but those are other dragons which we may perhaps meet on another occasion.

Sooner or later, we are going to have to come to terms with developing a common taxonomy. The use of multiple and eclectic frameworks for practice, classification systems that do not cover the full spectrum of nursing activities and inconsistent ways of documenting nursing practice hinder the design of nursing information systems. This is not to imply that there should be a common framework, but a common language is essential. There is more to identifying the domain of nursing than the relatively simple 'where does our turf begin and end' quandary. If we do not care for 'nursing diagnoses' we must engage in serious negotiating in a very short time. The world has shrunk since the days of Columbus, and is far too small a place for nursing research in any country to stand in isolation – but perhaps that is another frontier! And perhaps I am too hasty.

There is some evidence (Cohen, 1981; Corcoran, 1986; Hayes-Roth et al., 1983; Graves and Corcoran, 1989) which suggests that physicians and nurses structure their knowledge differently; generic problem solving skills are not necessarily those in common use. What is emerging is that expertise in human beings 'depends on domain knowledge and task-specific strategies' rather than on generic problem-solving strategies. Teaching students to utilise the 'nursing process' method of problem solving without the domain-specific knowledge is clearly inadequate.

The action statements for research within the Strategy document are worth repeating:

'1. Research awareness within the profession should be fostered. The teaching and application of research based knowledge to practice should be promoted.

2. Provision should be made for a number of experienced nurses to undertake research and opportunities afforded for postgraduate research and obtaining research degrees.

3. Direct research into clinical nursing issues should begin in the ward itself or at field level in the community.

4. Support should be given to nursing research units which should be effectively linked to higher education.

5. Consideration should be given to joint research appointments.

6. A database on Nursing Research should be set up.

7. Sources of funding for Nursing Research should be identified.

8. Links between Nursing Research Units and Ethical Committees must be established.'

DHSS, 1991

That should keep us busy for a time.

Nursing management

Statement 1 under the Management Strategy combines both leadership and management and focuses our attention for this frontier. It states that:

'There is a need for strong and effective nurse leadership and management if nurses are to adapt to the many and varied changes in the provision of health and social care proposed for the future in *Working for Patients, People First, Promoting Better Health, General Practice in the NHS – the 1990 Contract* and *Health Service Development.'*   DHSS, 1991

The management dragon

Our final dragon, (The Keeper of the Research-Based Practice Environment) is the *Management Dragon.*

Given the rapid and radical changes in the NHS at the present time, there is little familiar territory. Nurses in management and leadership positions are facing totally new challenges; senior nurses are out there adventuring this very minute. Certainly in Northern Ireland the frontiers are yet to be described. How might the future boundaries of nursing management show when mapped?

Features of high quality, cost-effective nursing care delivery systems of the future will be organised in clusters: delivery, evaluation, policy and marketing related characteristics are those which will be most prominent.

The features that affect the circumstances under which quality nursing services are provided are similar to those in the 'Magnet Hospitals' study of Kramer and

Schmalenberg (1988), based on the characteristics identified by Peters and Waterman (1982) in their famous book *In Search of Excellence*.

Delivery related features

Working relationships among nurses, physicians and other members of the health care team will facilitate the delivery of nursing services.

The organisation will attract and retain nurses with requisite clinical and management skills. Professional practice models that incorporate authority, autonomy, and responsibility – and at the same time offering appropriate compensation – will be a powerful incentive to both recruitment and retention. The time must come when practice roles are based on educational preparation and experience. Nursing, when we have defined both our activities (role) and domain (turf) will severely limit the use of professional time in clerical, housekeeping and maintenance tasks. We focus a great deal on what a profession is; we might do well to slay the *Do Everything Dragon*, which perpetuates our image of maid or domestic, and do what other professionals do – delegate non-professional activities to non-professionals.

The organisation will be characterised by sound financial planning, management, reporting, and *results*. Implicit are some key supports: nursing research focused on delivery of care, cost, outcomes, relationships to health care delivery in the broad sense, productivity data, efficiency data, and quality indicators related to cost.

Evaluation related features

Key evaluation related features follow logically. The organisation demonstrates cost effectiveness. Nurses providing services are accountable to consumers and are evaluated on the basis of care provided, in addition to their accountability to the employing organisation. Hancock, in a paper on the UK strategy for nursing (1990) claims that quality assurance is central to the nursing role. 'Survival of nursing leadership in the National Health Service will depend upon the response of individual nurses to the challenge of quality.' Furthermore, she asserts: 'If patient's expectations are low, and too often they are pitifully low, then it is certainly possible for a patient to be satisfied despite having received poor care. Objectively however, it is impossible for a hospital patient to have received quality care unless the nursing care was good.'

Policy related features

Policy related features refer to those features that affect nursing's ability to influence overall policies in organisations, hospitals or communities where nurses provide services. Nurses educated as they are now being educated, to be autonomous, confident, and in time, truly expert practitioners, expect a voice in policy making in decisions affecting their domain. Nurses must be formally placed to influence policy formation and implementation relevant to the organisation as a whole. Nurses are accountable and require authority over the fiscal resources for nursing practice. Clearly, hospitals must be financially viable to continue to exist. Aiken (1987) warns however, the financing of hospitals should not be nursings' main concern. Over identification with the concerns of management and preoccupation with the day-to-day operation of the institution divert nurses' time, attention and perhaps even loyalties away from patients and away from the clinical challenges and common interests they share with other health care professionals.

Marketing related features

Marketing related features are the features that affect the demand for nursing services. Whatever the system of the future, it must be flexible and responsive to changing needs and programme or service relevance. Nursing services will be marketed in terms of consumer need. Marketing means demonstrating and publicising the unique services provided by nurses within the broader context of health care.

To date, only delivery of nursing services is seen as clearly on our turf; I suspect evaluation of, policy making for and marketing our profession are areas often thought to be in forbidden territory, places to be avoided, beyond the dragons.

And how will nurses manage the delivery of the care of the future without resorting to the *Do Everything Dragon?* The best 'nurse extenders' are competent secretarial assistants and improved clinical computer systems. The number of nurses could be reduced without adversely affecting the care of patients if additional administrative, secretarial and clerical personnel were available to nurses. Nurses spend far more time than is necessary in organising care, coordinating services, transcribing orders, recording the work of others and documenting their own. (Aitken, 1987).

Who knows, some of these unexplored, undiscovered territories may yet resemble Utopia. There is adventure in practice, in education, in research and in management roles.

There is a price to pay for having this much fun. The concluding chapter in Peters and Austin's (1985) *A Passion for Excellence* was the starting point before this chapter was a gleam in a dragon's eye.

A passion for excellence means thinking big and starting small: excellence happens when high purpose and intense pragmatism meet. This is almost, but not quite, the whole truth. We believe a passion for excellence carries a price, and we state it simply: the adventure of excellence is not for the faint of heart.

Excellence and adventure are high cost items. Price any expedition. The price is time, energy, attention and focus; the rewards are commensurate – priceless.

References

Aiken, L.H. and Mullinix, C.F. (1987). The nurse shortage: myth or reality? *New England Journal of Medicine* 317: 641–46.

Barnett, J. (1974). The influence of community, in G. Collier *Values and moral development in higher education.* New York, John Wiley.

Benner, P. (1984). *From Novice to Expert: Excellence and Power in Clinical Nursing Practice*, Menlo Park, CA., Addison-Wesley.

Bevis, E.O. (1982). *Curriculum Building in Nursing*, St. Louis, CV Mosby.

Blinder, R. (1977). Moral development in higher education, *Image*, 9: 18–20.

Bosk, C.L. (1980). Occupational rituals in patient management, *New England Journal of Medicine*, 303: 71–76.

Brown, R. and Carron, H. (1978). Intentional moral development as an objective of higher education, *Journal of College Student Personnel*, 19: 426–429.

Brunner, L., Suddarth, D., Farics, B., Galligan, K., Lovoie, D. and Schwalenstoker, A. (1974). *The Lippincott Manual of Nursing Practice*, Philadelphia, Lippincott.

Carper, B.A. (1978). Fundamental patterns of knowing in nursing, *Advances in Nursing Science*, 1: 13–24.

Christman, L. (1976). Educational standards versus professional performance, in *Current Perspectives in Nursing Education: the Changing Scene*, St. Louis, CV Mosby.

Cohen, H.A. (1981). *The Nurses' Quest for a Professional Identity*, Menlo Park, CA., Addison-Wesley.

Corcoran, S. (1986). Planning by expert and novice nurses in cases of varying complexity, *Research in Nursing and Health*, 9: 155–162.

Dewey, J. (1909). *Moral Principles in Education*, Boston, Houghton-Mifflin.

DHSS (1991). *A Strategy for Nursing, Midwifery and Health Visiting in Northern Ireland*, Belfast, DHSS.

Emmerson, C. and Taylor, J. (1950). *Essentials of Medicine: the Basis of Nursing Care*, Philadelphia, Lippincott.

Fox, R.C., Aiken, L.H., and Messikomer, C.M. (1990). The culture of caring: AIDS and the nursing profession, *The Milbank Quarterly*, 68: 226–256.

Graves, J.R. and Corcoran, S. (1989) The study of nursing informatics, *Image*, 21(4): 227–231.

Group, T.M., and Robert, J.I. (1974). Exorcising the ghosts of the Crimea, *Nursing Outlook*, 22(6): 368–372.

Hancock, C. (1990). Leading the Way, *Nursing Standard*, 5: 3-5.

Harmer, B. and Henderson, V. (1939). *Textbook of the Principles and Practice of Nursing*, New York, Macmillan.

Hayes-Roth, F., Waterman, D. and Lenat, D. (eds). (1983). *Building Expert Systems*, New York, Addison-Wesley.

Holzemer, W. (1991). Editorial. *The Science of Caring*, 2: 1.

Kohlberg, L. (1976) The cognitive-developmental approach to moral education, in D. Purpel and K. Ryan (eds) *Moral Education: it comes with the Territory*, Berkeley, CA., McCutchon Publishing.

Kohlberg, L. (1978). The moral atmosphere of the school, in P. Scharf (ed) *Readings in Moral Education*, Minneapolis, Winston Press.

Kramer, M. (1974). *Reality Shock: Why Nurses Leave Nursing*, St. Louis, CV Mosby.

Kramer, M. and Chinn, P.L. (1988). Perspectives on knowing: a model of nursing knowledge, *Scholarly Inquiry in Nursing Practice*, 2: 129–139.

Kramer, M. and Schmalenberg, C. (1988). Magnet hospitals: institutions of excellence, *Journal of Nursing Administration*, 18: 11–19.

Livingstone, R. (1958). Plato and the training of character, *Educational Forum*, 23: 5–13.

O'Toole, A.W. and Loomis, M.A. (1989). Revision of the phenomena of concern for psychiatric mental health nursing, *Archives of Psychiatric Nursing*, 3: 288–299.

Peters, T.J. and Waterman, R.H. (1982) *In Search of Excellence*, New York, Harper and Row.

Peters, T. and Austin, N. (1985). *A Passion for Excellence*, Glasgow, William Collins.

Platt, J. (1980). The greatest evolutionary jump in history, in F. Feather and A. Toffer, (eds), *The Third Wave Through the 80s*, Washington, World Future Society.

Rogers, M. (1970). *An Introduction to the Theoretical Basis of Nursing*, Philadelphia, FA Davis.

Trow, M. (1976). Higher education and moral development, *AAUP Bulletin*, 62: 20–27.

Vito, K.O. (1983). Moral development considerations in nursing curricula, *Journal of Nursing Education*, 22: 108–113.

Wolf, Z.R. (1988). *Nurses' Work: the Sacred and the Profane*, Philadelphia, University of Pennsylvania Press.

Zadek, L.A. (1978). A fuzzy algorithmic approach to the definition of complex or imprecise concepts, *International journal of Man-Machine Studies*, 8: 249–291.

Index